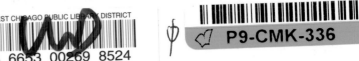

How to Teach Nutrition to Kids

4th Edition

Connie Liakos Evers, MS, RD

24 Carrot Press ◆ Portland, Oregon

24 Carrot Press
P.O. Box 23546
Portland, OR 97281
503-524-9318
www.nutritionforkids.com

The information, suggestions and activities contained in this book are not intended, nor should anything contained herein be construed as, an attempt to give, or be a substitute for, medical advice or medical nutrition therapy. Individuals with specific food or nutrition needs, such as, but not limited to, food allergies and/or intolerances, should not rely solely on information, suggestions or activities contained in this book. Such individuals should be evaluated and treated by qualified health professionals.

Cover Design & Illustration: Carol Buckle, www.cjbuckle.com

Printed in the United States of America

ISBN: 978-0-9647970-0-0

Library of Congress Control Number: 2012930168

More books by Connie Liakos Evers, MS, RD
> Nutrition Fun with Brocc & Roll, 2nd ed. (24 Carrot Press, ©2012)
> Good for You! Nutrition Book and Games (Disney Press, ©2006)

For updates, free resources and more, visit us online:
> www.nutritionforkids.com
> www.facebook.com/nutritionforkids
> twitter.com/nutritionkids

On the Cover: The Nutrition for Kids foodies line up in accordance with the *MyPlate* food guidance system.

To Mom and Dad,
Thank you for teaching me about
cooking, nutrition, gardening
and the importance of family meals.

Acknowledgements

Gratitude is the word that comes to mind when I contemplate how this book continues to be a useful resource for so many. In the beginning, I nervously anticipated that a few teachers and perhaps some dietitians might be interested. I never imagined that the book would be useful to such a diverse audience. Besides schools, the book is used by health care professionals, chefs, scout leaders, parents, grandparents, summer camps, YMCA programs, health departments, cooperative extension, WIC and just about any program that serves youth. Most surprising to me are the dozens of colleges and universities that use *How to Teach Nutrition to Kids* as a text or supplementary text in school health and nutrition courses.

To every teacher, leader, parent, professor and student, I thank you all.

I am also in gratitude to all who helped me along the way. As I made the revisions, it saddened me that I have lost contact with many of the professionals that influenced this book: teachers Carolyn Johnson, Adele White, and Jennifer Butler as well as Chef Gordon MacDonald come to mind.

Thank you to the students of Beaverton and Portland schools who wrote funny, endearing and often revealing thank you letters over the years, some of which are excerpted in the quotes that begin each chapter.

I'm appreciative of Carol Buckle, graphic designer and friend who, in addition to her wonderful cover design and illustrations, always makes me laugh.

I'm indebted to the many professionals who have helped and inspired me along the way: Bob Honson; Brenda Ponichtera, RD; Bridget Swinney, MS, RD; Penny Price, MS; Sandy Miller, MS, RD; Anita Kobuszewski, MS, RD; Vickie James, RD; Carolyn Morrison. I'm also grateful to my dear, late friend Margaret Raker, a teacher, dietitian and attorney, who left this earth far too soon.

Finally, I'm grateful for the support and love from Scott, Kelli, Sam and Adam.

Contents

Introduction

" My hope is that children will learn to enjoy a variety of healthful foods, find pleasure in physical activity and feel satisfaction in their growing, developing bodies." —CLE

I have been a nutrition educator for nearly thirty years. During this time, I have witnessed a great deal of discussion, debate and advocacy aimed at improving the nutrition and health environment for children. While the statistics for child obesity and other health indicators are alarming, I have also seen a renewed and urgent action-oriented focus on child health, particularly in the past five years. Nutrition for children is now a hot button issue, with involvement from many sectors, including government, education, academia, nonprofits, the media and industry. I'm optimistic that by working together, we may finally make some headway in improving the health of our most precious resource, our children.

The purpose of this book is to provide educators, health care professionals, parents and other caregivers with hands-on tools as well as the inspiration they need to teach 5- to 12-year-old children about food and nutrition in a fun, meaningful and integrated way.

Many of the ideas are drawn from my experience as a nutrition educator working with thousands of students in schools as well as my most cherished role as a parent of three children. Along the way, I have learned a great deal about how to succeed in teaching nutrition to kids and guiding them towards positive health behaviors. I have also had a lot of fun doing it! I hope you share my enthusiasm and allow your own creativity to expand and build on the many ideas presented here.

Connie Liakos Evers, MS, RD
March 2012

How to Use This Book

A cooperative approach among caregivers is necessary if children are to both learn and practice good eating habits. Described below are suggestions on how those who care for and teach children can best incorporate ideas and activities from this book.

Educators

The chapters in this book bear little resemblance to a standard nutrition book. Take a look at the Table of Contents. Instead of chapters like Vegetables, Vitamins or Weight Control, you will see Language Arts, Math, Science and Social Studies, the subjects teachers spend time on *every* day of the school year. Many of the lesson ideas are designed with time in mind — easy to implement with little preparation. Others can be modified for simplicity or expanded into a comprehensive unit. For instance, the gardening ideas in Chapter 7 could easily comprise a year-long theme.

Throughout this book, you can readily identify how nutrition lesson ideas cross over into other disciplines. The following picture symbols identify related subject areas:

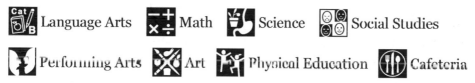 Language Arts   Math   Science   Social Studies
Performing Arts   Art   Physical Education   Cafeteria

Activities that require materials and supplies beyond what is commonly found in most classrooms are highlighted with "You Will Need" boxes. Activities are categorized according to level (Primary, Intermediate or Either) in the index listing for each subject area.

Chapter 4, "Teaching the Basics of Healthful Eating," provides guidance on how to design your introductory nutrition unit, ideally taught early in the school year. Once students have a grasp of these basic concepts, you can expand and reinforce nutrition by integrating it into your curriculum throughout the year. As you plan your units of instruction and learning centers, keep this book handy. Refer to each subject area chapter as you plan lessons.

Many of the nutrition ideas may be the hook to get kids motivated in other subjects, too. Writing a letter to "Baby Bear," graphing food intake or analyzing the school lunch menu can make writing, math and critical thinking more exciting and relevant.

Before you plan lessons involving food preparation, please review Appendix A, "Guidelines for Safe Classroom Cooking."

Finally, take a look around your classroom. Are food and nutrition teaching materials up to date? If you have a kitchen, grocery store or restaurant as part of your dramatic play area, do the play foods include mostly healthful choices? An inexpensive way to update this area is to use actual food packages such as beans and brown rice, empty boxes, cartons and stuffed whole grain bread wrappers. For colorful fruit and vegetable models, cut out photos from gardening catalogs and grocery flyers and glue onto foam core.

Resources for low-cost materials that will brighten your classroom and reinforce nutrition concepts are listed in Appendix B.

Food/Nutrition Professionals

In nearly every chapter, students are encouraged to become involved with the school nutrition program. Examples include forming student advisory groups, hosting tours of the school kitchen, encouraging open communication with the school nutrition director, analyzing the school breakfast and lunch menus and performing lunchtime nutrition skits.

Just as nutrition is integrated into all subject areas, this book also gives guidance for integrating nutrition education into the school meal program. After all, the school cafeteria is the ultimate laboratory, giving students the chance to practice nutrition concepts each day.

Whenever possible, make yourself available to the teachers and students in your school. Volunteer to be a guest speaker on nutrition. Your presentation can be as simple as reading a storybook with a good-food message or as complicated as setting up a classroom sandwich bar to illustrate a meal that exemplifies the *MyPlate* Food Guide. This book provides hundreds of ideas on classroom nutrition lessons.

Another powerful way to reinforce nutrition concepts is to run promotions in the cafeteria. Menu or recipe contests, food-of-the-week displays, nutrition bingo with small incentives, student poster art and point-of-choice nutrition information encourage students to make healthful food choices. Chapter 12 provides guidance on how to turn the cafeteria into a center for nutrition education.

Parents

You are the ultimate gatekeeper of nutrition. What you buy, how you cook and the foods that *you* eat or refuse all send strong messages about food to your child. The best way to educate your child about nutrition and health is to model good eating behavior.

Beyond your role as food provider and living example, there are many other ways to teach your child about food and nutrition. A number of ideas in this book can easily be adapted for learning situations in the home. Tending a small garden plot, reading and discussing books with nutrition messages or using the grocery store as a learning center are just a few examples.

Involve your child in the kitchen. It is true that cooking with your child may add to the time, mess and confusion initially. But eventually, you will appreciate both the extra set of hands and your child's growing self-sufficiency.

Many of the food activities, especially the edible art creations in Chapter 10, work well in group settings such as birthday parties, scout meetings or large family gatherings.

This book can also serve as a stepping stone for initiating a nutrition education program in your local elementary school. Activities and ideas can be implemented by parent volunteers in the classroom or at school wellness, health, multicultural or science fairs. Information presented here also provides valuable guidance for setting school nutrition policy.

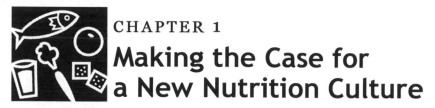

CHAPTER 1

Making the Case for a New Nutrition Culture

"As parents and educators, it is our job to create a new culture for health, one where we model good eating and fitness habits, provide healthy shared meals and set limits on foods with little nutritional value." –CLE

A Great Need

Children today face an increasing number of nutrition problems, including fragmented eating habits, poor food choices, obesity and eating disorders. We are obviously failing to create an environment that is conducive to healthy eating and lifetime physical activity. Current findings shed a dim light on the state of children's eating and exercise habits.

OBESITY

Findings from the National Health and Nutrition Examination Survey (NHANES) reveal a staggering increase in childhood obesity since 1976. Between 1976 and 2008, the prevalence of childhood obesity increased:

- From 5.0% to 10.4% among 2–5 year olds
- From 6.5% to 19.6% among 6–11 year olds
- From 5.0% to 18.1% among 12-19 year olds

Not only do obese children face an uncertain future health picture, they are at risk right now for the debilitating effects of extra weight, such as high blood cholesterol levels and high blood pressure, which are risk factors for cardiovascular disease. Obesity also increases the risk of impaired glucose tolerance, insulin resistance and type 2 diabetes as well as asthma, sleep apnea, joint problems and digestive difficulties such as gastro-esophageal reflux. Obese children and adolescents are also at higher risk of social and psychological problems, such as poor self-esteem and discrimination. It is estimated that about half of obese school-agers and 70 percent of obese teens of will remain obese into adulthood.

This epidemic increase in childhood obesity is particularly prevalent among African American and Hispanic children and teens. For example, recent data show that among 12-19 year-olds, 29.2% of black girls and 26.8% of Mexican American boys meet the criteria for obesity.

INACTIVITY

While the CDC and other organizations recommend that children participate in physical activity a minimum of an hour daily, kids are actually engaging in *less* physical activity, particularly as they approach adolescence. One study documented a severe drop in physical activity between the ages of 9 and 15. Nearly half of American youths ages 12–21 are not vigorously active on a regular basis.

A big contributor to this trend is our fixation on all things electronic. Kids spend large chunks of passive time in front of screens such as television, cell phones, video games, tablets and computers. Studies have documented a connection between the time spent watching TV and body fat percentage in children. Screen time in all its forms has replaced active play time for many kids and teens.

POOR FOOD CHOICES

With a food supply as plentiful and varied as we have in the United States, it is shocking to note the dismal state of children's (and adults') food habits. The majority of both children and adults have a diet that falls into the category of "needs improvement," according to the Healthy Eating Index-2005 (HEI-2005), a scale that measures 12 components of a healthy diet. On a scale of 100, children's scores average just 59.6 for preschoolers and 54.7 and 54.8 for ages 6-11 and 2-17, respectively.

In particular, kids need to eat more whole fruit, whole grains, legumes and dark green and orange vegetables. Over half of the vegetables currently eaten by children come from either potatoes (usually fried) or tomatoes. Data from the HEI-2005 also shows a need to limit saturated fat, sodium, and extra calories from solid fats and added sugars (SoFAS). According to the Dietary Guidelines for Americans, 2010, a shocking 35% of a typical American's calories come from SoFAS.

Few youngsters take in enough calcium to maximize their lifetime bone development. At a time when they need calcium the most, kids are choosing sugary drinks over dairy products. While recent government recommendations advise a calcium intake of 1,300 milligrams for children ages 9-18, nutrition surveys show a decline in calcium intake for this age group, with fewer than half consuming the recommended amount each day. Low-fat or fat-free dairy products are a major source of several nutrients, including calcium, vitamin D, and potassium, which are identified as "nutrients of concern" in the Dietary Guidelines for Americans, 2010. For children who are allergic to dairy or follow a vegan diet, it is important to include calcium fortified soy or other plant-based beverages.

"Americans eat too many calories and too much solid fat, added sugars, refined grains, and sodium. Americans also consume too little potassium; dietary fiber; calcium; vitamin D; unsaturated fatty acids from oils, nuts, and seafood; and other important nutrients. These nutrients are mostly found in vegetables, fruits, whole grains, and low-fat milk and milk products."
Source: Dietary Guidelines for Americans, 2010 Policy Report

While snacking can contribute important nutrients to a child's diet, studies show that snacks are often a source of high-calorie, low-nutrient foods such as sugary beverages, fried chips, grain-based desserts and sweet snacks. Total daily calorie intake from snacks among children has risen from an average of 450 to 600 calories per day since the late 1970s, according to researchers at the University of North Carolina at Chapel Hill.

PORTIONS OUT OF CONTROL

It's no coincidence that we've seen a dramatic increase in the size of both food portions and our waistlines in recent years. At fast food restaurants, so-called "value" meals offer little value to our health and well-being. For just a few more cents, we can stuff in an excess of mostly empty-calorie food and sugary beverages.

It's not just our imaginations — researchers have documented that the size of most food portions are increasing. Data from government surveys show that portion sizes in both restaurants *and* at home are increasing at an alarming rate. Even our plates, bowls and glasses have increased in size over the past 30 years.

Simply put, larger servings translate into more calories. Researchers have shown that even as early as the preschool years, children will eat more when presented with larger portions.

SUGARY BEVERAGES

"Got sweetened beverages?" seems to be the real slogan for today's kids. Over the past thirty years, guzzling of sugary beverages has soared among children while intake of milk has declined. This tendency to pick sweet drinks over more nutritious beverages actually begins in the early pre-school years. By adolescence, nearly one in four teens drinks more than 26 ounces of soft drinks daily.

One study documented that when children consumed an average of 9 ounces of soft drinks daily, their total daily calories increased, while key nutrients such as folate, vitamin A, vitamin C and calcium took a nosedive.

These liquid calories are not just coming from soft drinks — there has been a tremendous increase in other sweetened beverage choices. Grocery store shelves overflow with bottles of sweetened fruit drinks, teas, sports beverages and more recently, energy drinks. The American Academy of Pediatrics released a report in 2011 stating that in most cases, kids rarely need sports drinks, and that energy drinks are never appropriate for children or adolescents, as some of these products contain caffeine and other substances that could be harmful to children. The report also urges parents to serve water to rehydrate and low-fat or fat-free milk to help hydrate and meet nutrient needs.

HUNGRY CHILDREN

How can the same overnourished nation described here possibly have people who go hungry? It is shocking but true that hunger and inadequate nutrition continue to impact a startling number of children in America. A government report released in 2011 indicates that nearly ten percent of households with children are considered "food insecure," meaning they do not always have access to enough food for active, healthy lives for all household members.

Hungry children often fail to achieve their full academic potential. Children with inadequate diets are sick more, less active, less able to think and concentrate and more irritable and anxious. In one study, 6- to 11-year-old food-insufficient children had lower arithmetic scores and were more likely to have repeated a grade, have seen a psychologist and have had difficulty getting along with other children. Kids with iron deficiency anemia score lower on IQ tests (especially in vocabulary) and suffer from perceptual difficulties and low achievement.

Though it may seem counterintuitive, children in food insecure households are also at risk for obesity. Lack of access to healthy, affordable foods, fewer opportunities for physical activity and limited access to health care all contribute to childhood obesity, according to the Food Research and Action Center.

One partial solution to this problem is better promotion of the school breakfast and lunch programs. Regardless of income level, children who eat school meals have higher intakes of key nutrients and perform better in school.

Opportunity for Change

The news about children's health is not all bad. On the upside, a tremendous amount of interest, effort and opportunity currently surrounds this problem.

THE POWER OF PARENTS

Parents still have considerable influence over the eating patterns of their children. Studies point to a strong association between parents who model good nutrition and improved eating habits in their youngsters.

Family meals provide tremendous benefits to the health and well-being of children. Kids and teens who eat meals with their families on a more frequent basis have higher intakes of vegetables, calcium-rich food, fiber, calcium, magnesium, potassium, iron, zinc, folate, and vitamins A and B6. According to research from Project EAT (Eating Among Teens) at the University of Minnesota, family meals are also related to higher academic performance, greater psychosocial well-being and a reduced risk of unhealthy weight control behaviors.

Parents are also important partners in their children's nutrition education outside of the home. School-based nutrition programs that involve parents are more effective at changing children's eating behaviors than those that focus solely on the student.

KIDS IN THE KITCHEN

As children become more self-reliant at an earlier age, a "teachable moment" exists for strengthening food-related life skills.

Children who don't know how to cook tend to rely on fast foods or convenience foods of questionable nutritional quality. For this growing number of young consumers, nutrition education can really work when concepts are practical and applied, emphasizing skills such as shopping, label reading and cooking. Kids who are on their own for meals can immediately translate their nutrition knowledge into healthy eating behavior.

SCHOOL MEALS

Schools who participate in the United States Department of Agriculture (USDA) child nutrition program are required to serve meals that meet the Dietary Guidelines for Americans. The Healthy, Hunger-Free Kids Act of 2010 strengthens nutrition standards and also gives USDA the authority to set nutritional standards for all foods regularly sold in schools during the school day, including vending machines, the "a la carte" lunch lines and school stores.

While many schools throughout the nation have made progress towards offering healthier school meals, there are still a number of barriers to overcome, including limited resources, outdated facilities, and at times, resistance from both staff and students. Chapter 12 offers successful strategies for transforming the cafeteria environment and serving nutritious, kid-appealing meals.

EDUCATION

When educators realize that well-nourished students learn better, they are more inclined to move beyond merely teaching the food groups and instead teach nutrition in a comprehensive, behavior-oriented manner.

A report from the National Center for Education Statistics found that while 88 percent of elementary school teachers reported teaching nutrition in the classroom, not nearly enough time was devoted to nutrition education during the year. The mean number of hours spent on nutrition instruction was 13, well below the 50 hours thought to be necessary for impact on behavior.

Success at classroom nutrition education requires that teachers have sufficient background, training, resources and, of course, the time to teach it all. One goal of this book is to aid teachers in integrating nutrition across the curriculum and into the daily lives of students.

A Call to Action

Clearly, the efforts of many are needed to reverse the trends set forth here. The messages children receive about nutrition should be clear, consistent and constant. Only then will kids begin to internalize the information and make changes in their eating and activity habits. This formidable task of creating a healthy food culture is shared by all who influence kids' food choices: parents, extended family, educators, coaches, food/nutrition professionals, health care providers, researchers, the food industry, the media, government agencies and legislators.

Most important, the food available to children must match the messages they are hearing. Whether at school, home, the ballpark or a restaurant, healthy choices that appeal to kids are essential. Kids don't get proficient at playing the piano, solving math problems or scoring soccer goals without a lot of practice — the same is true of good nutrition habits!

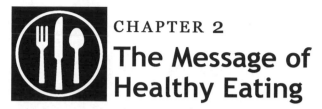

CHAPTER 2

The Message of Healthy Eating

"If we are to instill healthy attitudes about food and body image in our children, we must start early, presenting a unified message about food as fuel and bodies as something to be proud of and happy about." –CLE

Finding a Balance

MEDIA MESSAGES

Presenting a balanced picture of nutrition is no easy task in today's society. The media confuses us daily, reporting the latest nutrition study as fact, leaving us dazed as we contemplate whether our favorite foods have been praised or denounced this week. We quickly lose sight of the fact that food is an integral part of life that should be savored and enjoyed.

Likewise, children are sent a mind-boggling set of mixed messages from television, social networking sites, websites and print media. On one hand, kids see mostly attractive people — at least by Hollywood or Madison Avenue's standard — who are thin, rich, popular and fun-loving. On the other hand, they are barraged with advertisements for foods with little nutritional value. When they do see models, actors and celebrities eating, it is usually in ads or placed endorsements that peddle empty calorie foods such as candy, fried snacks, fast food and soft drinks.

Beginning at a young age, kids are bombarded by advertising messages. In addition to the thousands of television ads each year aimed directly at the youth market, companies also reach children through product placements, licensing of popular characters, viral buzz through social networking sites and mobile devices, in-school promotions, online "advergames," kids' clubs and many other strategies.

> **Plugged In Kids**
> A 2010 report from the Kaiser Family Foundation found that 8-18 year-olds devote an average of over 53 hours per week to entertainment media and they often use several devices at once. Almost two-thirds of the kids surveyed reported that television was usually on during mealtime.
> *Source: Generation M2: Media in the Lives of 8- to 18-Year-Olds*
> *http://www.kff.org/entmedia/8010.cfm*

Food and beverages are the most advertised products on television programming aimed at kids. According to the report, *Food for thought: Television food advertising to children in the United States,* kids and teens see an average of 4400 to 7600 food ads per year, yet they see fewer than 165 ads that promote fitness or good nutrition.

Most of the foods advertised contain excess fat, sugar or sodium (or a combination of the three) and provide little nutritional value. In 2009, the fast-food industry alone spent $4.2 billion on advertising in all media. Adding to the confusion, many ads directed at kids are deceptive in their nature. For instance, breakfast cereals, candy-like snacks and sugary beverages with "fruit" or "fruity" in their names are depicted in ads that include colorful images of real fruit. In actuality, many of the products contain no fruit or juice, relying on artificial flavors and colors for their "fruitiness."

While advertisers may be satisfied to know that their messages are working, the ultimate outcome of their efforts is detrimental to children's health. Studies show that there is a direct association between the number of hours of television viewed and the number of requests from children to buy the products they see advertised. Kids who watch the most TV have higher intakes of calories, fat, fried snacks, sweets and soft drinks and lower intakes of fruits and vegetables.

Even the youngest children are being swayed by marketers. In an experiment to test the impact of television commercials on the food preferences of 2- to 6-year-olds, researchers found that brief embedded commercials in a cartoon videotape directly influenced the preschoolers' food choices.

ALTERED BODY IMAGE

Not only is our society getting fatter, we also feel more guilty about it, a feeling children are acquiring at an alarmingly young age. In a study of 10- and 11-year-old Girls Scouts, 29 percent of the girls were trying to lose weight. More than 60 percent of fourth grade girls in an Iowa study reported a desire to be thinner. By age 18, nine out of ten teenage girls in a California survey were dieting to lose weight.

This perception of fatness is common even among girls with little body fat. In one study, 58 percent of girls ages 9 to 18 thought of themselves as fat, whereas only 15 percent were overweight based on height and weight measures. Fear of fatness, restrained eating and binge eating were found to be common among girls by age 10.

Boys are not immune to body image issues and disordered eating behaviors. In addition to restrained eating and excessive exercise, they may also engage in unhealthy practices (e.g. steroids and unsafe dietary supplements) that they believe will result in a more muscular physique.

Parents have a powerful influence on their children's self-esteem and body image. Researchers found that measured self-esteem scores of kids ages 9–11 were lowered when they thought their parents were dissatisfied with their bodies. In boys, a lowered self-esteem was linked with both thinness and being perceived as too thin by parents. Not surprisingly, lowered self-esteem in girls had more to do with parental attitudes toward fatness. In one study, moms who constantly diet directly influence their 5-year-old daughters' ideas about dieting.

> **Reading Magazines Can be Harmful to Your Health**
> In a five year study of teen girls, the odds of engaging in unhealthy weight-control behaviors (such as fasting, skipping meals, and smoking more cigarettes) were twice as high for the girls who read the most magazine articles about dieting and weight loss.
> Source: van den Berg, P., Neumark-Sztainer, D., Hannan, P., & Haines, J. (2007). Is dieting advice from magazines helpful or harmful? Pediatrics, 119(1), e30-e37.

Adding to the image problem is a small but worrisome group of overzealous parents. Determined that their child will not be fat or eat fat, they restrict food intake starting at a very young age. Kids who comply with their parents' wishes often end up underweight and at risk for delayed growth. Those who rebel may end up overweight because they have a tendency to overeat whenever they get the chance.

There is a wide variation in growth patterns and rates among kids. Children of the same age can vary as much as 40 pounds and 10 inches and still be considered normal by typical growth standards. Unfortunately, kids don't see a wide variety of shapes and sizes depicted in magazines or television. Even their school textbooks carry a size bias. An analysis of third-grade texts since the beginning of the century found that illustrations of girls became increasingly thinner through the years, while no change was noted for pictures of boys.

Creating Positive Attitudes

Reversing the trend of feeling guilty about food and weight, resulting in indulgence, more weight and more guilt, can only be arrested through education and self awareness.

If we are to instill healthy attitudes about food and body image in our children, we must start early, presenting a unified message about food as fuel and bodies as something to be proud of and happy about.

Now the hard part: we, as adult role models, must reach some degree of satisfaction with ourselves! Women, in particular, spend enormous amounts of time and energy pursuing an elusive ideal of a perfect body. In our constant obsession to diet, exercise and engage in dubious weight loss practices, we often forget that our basic body shape was predetermined at birth.

It's no wonder we're confused. In our lifetime alone, we have seen the ideal female body form go from voluptuous to outright undernourished. In an analysis of Miss America Pageant winners, researchers observed a drop in the Body Mass Index (BMI) over time. Only 23 percent of the winners had a BMI in the normal range of 20–25, and 26 percent actually met the World Health Organization's definition of undernourished (BMI < 18.5).

WHAT WE CAN DO

Despite the influence of popular culture, there are steps we can take to instill healthy attitudes in our children:

▲ Affirm children. When kids complain about being too fat, skinny, short, tall or slow, emphasize the goodness about them. Assure kids that people come in all different colors, shapes and sizes. Every child has a unique pattern of growth and will enter growth spurts at different times. Remind kids that there is no one "best" way to look.

▲ Children who you suspect are overweight should be referred to a qualified health care provider for evaluation and treatment. Often, counseling of an overweight child requires cooperation and participation by the entire family and school community.

▲ Emphasize the enjoyable aspects of food. Avoid labeling food as either medicine or poison. With older children especially, telling them "it's good for you" may actually discourage healthful eating habits. Likewise, kids are not immediately concerned that a food they like may clog their arteries or decay their teeth. Scare tactics rarely work.

▲ Children should have a choice over their eating and control over their bodies. Given a selection of healthful foods, kids have an amazing ability to self-regulate their diet. In spite of good intentions, adults impair the development of normal eating habits when they attempt to control a child's food intake.

Taken to extremes, an over controlling parent places a child at risk for developing eating disorders such as obesity, bulimia and anorexia nervosa.

Parents' Actions, Not Words, Key to Better Nutrition for Kids

If parents ate more fruits and vegetables, so did their daughters, researchers found in a study of 200 5-year-old girls and their parents. Parents who pressured their daughters the most about eating fruits and vegetables were those who consumed the least of these foods. Their daughters ate 1.6 fewer servings of fruits and vegetables a day than the daughters of parents who used less pressure. The researchers recommend that parents set a good example by eating plenty of fruits and vegetables and by not nagging.

Source: Fisher, J., Mitchell, D., Smiciklas-Wright, H., & Birch, L. (2002). Parental influences on young girls' fruit and vegetable, micronutrient, and fat intakes. Journal of The American Dietetic Association, 102(1), 58-64.

▲ Encourage children to move play and exercise, both at home and at school. Besides physical education and recess time, kids (and teachers, too) can benefit from discovery classroom walks (see Chapter 11).

At home, kids will gravitate toward more activity if they are regularly unplugged from television, mobile devices, computers and video games. Parents also reap benefits from family walks, bike rides, games and other shared activities.

▲ Make mealtime a priority. Breaking bread together promotes good nutrition habits. School-aged children who eat alone in front of the television tend to overeat, while younger children tend to eat fewer nutritious foods when isolated at meals.

Mealtime means more than refueling kids with nutrients — they also get a hefty dose of emotional, intellectual and spiritual nourishment. As families pass the peas and pour the milk, they also convey values and establish traditions.

Pay attention to the school mealtime atmosphere, too. Work to improve nutrition, taste, presentation and the overall mealtime atmosphere at school. Bright cafeterias, short lines and adequate time for children to eat should be goals of every school. Kids should be allowed to relax and socialize — these skills are also components of learning and development. Schools with limited facilities may want to explore family-style eating in the classroom.

What Kids Need to Know

Clearly, children are in need of balanced, sensible messages about eating and nutrition. An important goal of nutrition education is to enlighten and empower kids so they will grow to be adults who make informed food choices and avoid the lure of food fads and nutrition hype.

What then, should we be teaching kids? The following points outline the basic goals of nutrition education for kids. Chapters 4–12 provide specific, hands-on activities for reaching these goals.

▲ Emphasize food as it relates to life today. You will lose kids' attention faster than they can say osteoporosis if too much emphasis is placed on how proper nutrition prevents disease. If you succeed in reaching them with the good nutrition message today, their tomorrows will likely be healthier, too.

Remind children that healthful food promotes achievement. In school or on the playing field, kids who eat well perform better and achieve higher levels of mastery. A nutritious diet fuels the body for learning, growth, sports and play.

Well-nourished kids also look healthy. Children who eat a balanced diet have eyes that sparkle, skin that glows and bodies that are fit and energetic.

▲ The message of good nutrition is summed up in the Dietary Guidelines for Americans (DGA), 2010. The DGA emphasize three major goals for Americans:

- Balance calories with physical activity to manage weight.

- Consume more of certain foods and nutrients such as fruits, vegetables, whole grains, fat-free and low-fat dairy products, and seafood.

- Consume fewer foods with sodium, saturated fats, trans fats, cholesterol, added sugars, and refined grains.

Revised every five years, the Dietary Guidelines for Americans are designed to help Americans choose diets that will meet nutrient requirements, promote health, support active lives and reduce the risk of chronic disease. The DGA also form the basis for U.S. food policies that affect nutrition programs such as the USDA School Meals, summer and after school food programs, the child and adult care food program (CACFP), the Special Nutrition Assistance Program (SNAP, formerly known as food stamps), and the Supplemental Food Program for Women, Infants and Children (WIC). For more information about the research behind the 2010 DGA as well as resources and educational materials, visit DietaryGuidelines.gov.

Two important practical tools for meeting the 2010 DGA are the *MyPlate* food guide and the *Nutrition Facts* food label. An icon that represents the image of a healthy diet, *MyPlate* is especially useful as a teaching aid for children. The *Nutrition Facts* label is a simplified, yet effective, device for analyzing foods and comparing nutrient contents. Ideas for developing a nutrition unit around *MyPlate* and *Nutrition Facts* labels are included, respectively, in Chapters 4 and 6.

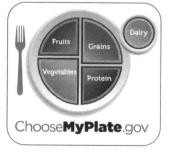

▲ Teach children to refuel their bodies with regular, nutritious meals and snacks. Because of their smaller stomach capacity and tremendous energy needs, kids require frequent meals and snacks. Behavior problems at times are merely the result of an empty stomach.

Breakfast is the meal most directly connected to school achievement. Kids who skip breakfast have a shorter attention span, do poorly in tasks requiring concentration and even score lower on standard achievement tests. There is also research that suggests breakfast eaters have an easier time achieving a healthy weight.

When researchers compared the diets of children who regularly eat breakfast with those who don't, they found that the breakfast skippers never fully compensate for the missed meal throughout the day. Children who ate a morning meal took in far more nutrients over the course of the day than those who missed breakfast. An optimal breakfast includes a protein source (from either the protein or dairy group), a serving of whole grain and a serving of either fruit or vegetable

Somehow, snacking has taken on a negative connotation in our society, perhaps because it is often linked with fried chips, sweet treats and other empty calorie foods. Done right, snacks can and do make a big contribution to daily nutrition. Healthy snacks should mirror meals — emphasizing nutritious foods from 2-3 different food groups, but in smaller quantities.

▲ Young bodies need to move. Kids should be getting at least one hour of moderate to vigorous physical activity each day. Ideally, they will spend additional time participating in active play and transportation. Nutrition studies show that the current epidemic of childhood obesity stems from both inactivity and overeating. An intricate balance exists between food and physical activity. A nutrition unit will be lacking if it fails to present the exercise part of the equation.

Kids enjoy learning about nutrition when it is presented from a fitness perspective. That's why Chapter 11 is devoted to nutrition as a component of the physical education curriculum. Physical fitness should also be part of the daily classroom routine, especially in schools that limit PE to once or twice weekly.

▲ Media literacy should be a part of every child's education, both at school and at home. If children are to resist the allure of the media, advertisements and other societal influences, they must learn to identify the intent of the messages. Even very young children can grasp the basic purpose of advertising (to sell us stuff). Older children will enjoy homework they really can do in front of the TV, i.e., analyze and critique food ads.

Role playing is a very effective way to teach children the messages of the media and encourage the development of critical thinking and decision-making skills. Chapter 9 outlines several strategies for helping children to analyze and re-create the food messages they hear each day from TV, radio, magazines and peers.

CHAPTER 3
The F.I.B. Approach to Nutrition Education

"Thank you for the very tasty lesson — and the good yogurt with blueberries, bananas, strawberries and granola. Combined to make a masterpiece." —Jeremy

There was little in my training to become a registered dietitian that prepared me to teach nutrition to kids. In college, I spent my time learning the scientific basis of nutrition and key principles of food management. Not that metabolic pathways, bowel transit time or hospital trayline efficiency weren't important issues, it's just that I failed to grasp the practical issues at the heart of feeding and teaching kids.

I wasn't sure what to do when my own children refused to eat, decorated the wall with spaghetti, nicknamed coconuts "dog poop balls" or stuffed peas up the nose. (*In case you are wondering, the correct answers are: Relax; Recognize the cue that your child is done eating; Ignore and try not to laugh; Call the pediatrician*)

And, early in my career, 1 was guilty of boring school kids to sleep by lecturing them about food groups and vitamins!

It was in my position as the nutrition education coordinator for a large urban school district that I gained valuable insight from those around me — teachers, coaches, parents, foodservice professionals and *especially* the students. I came to realize that key elements were often missing from successful efforts at nutrition education.

Boiled down to three words, the ingredients I discovered necessary for effective nutrition education with children are **Fun**, **Integrated** and **Behavioral**, or F.I.B. for short. This approach is supported by research as well as my personal experience in nutrition education.

Begin by Making It Fun!

Like it or not, today's kids are easily bored. They are constantly online and plugged in to various forms of electronic media, often interacting with several devices at once. Children and teens are used to information that is entertaining, fast-paced and exciting. In a word, "fun."

Teachers increasingly need to engage as well as educate students. While this approach can mean more planning, the payoff is a boost in motivation. Children who enjoy themselves through discovery and experimentation are much more apt to listen and retain information.

An added benefit is that educators who create engaging lessons often find more satisfaction in their jobs. Experiential activities involving food, role playing, music and movement are enjoyable for students as well as adult leaders and teachers. During my career as a nutrition educator, I have:

▲ Appeared in classrooms around Halloween as "Nutra the Witch," teaching kids how to make "food group brew," choose healthful snacks and limit their candy "goblin."

▲ Acted in noontime nutrition shows for elementary schools with two full-sized dog characters named Sheggy Good-Grub and Sickly Spot. Sheggy's nickname was SHEG, which is an acronym for the four things nutrition gives a young body — strength, health, energy and growth. I even led the cafeteria in a round of "The Sheggy Good-Grub Song," in spite of dubious vocal skills. (Once, it was even broadcast on CNN!)

▲ Used my own baby as a "visual aid." Frustrated with my inability to reach teen moms and educate them on proper nutrition and feeding development, I brought my 10-month-old son along to demonstrate techniques for infant feeding. My son loved the attention and the adolescent moms began paying attention to my lessons.

▲ Developed *Crazy for Veggies* and *Go Bananas for Fruit* kits consisting of interactive worksheets, stickers and tasting/preparation ideas in order to motivate children to include more fruits and vegetables in their diets.

▲ Sang, danced, exercised, cooked and led puppet shows with elementary school kids more times than I can count.

THINK BIG!

When planning a nutrition lesson or entire unit, brainstorm creative ways to make the concepts come alive. Say, for example, kids are routinely feeding their oranges to the trash during lunch. Your goal is to encourage kids to eat (or at least try) oranges.

Talking about oranges is boring. Putting up colorful posters of oranges throughout the school is a little better. Providing cut up oranges for snacks is better still.

But to really make an impact, declare one day "Orange Day." Serve orange juice on the breakfast menu and orange wedges at lunch. Encourage students, staff and visiting parents to wear orange, call the citrus commission to see if they have teaching materials (and maybe even an orange costume to lend) and set up centers where students can make orange juice, plant the seeds from their oranges or write a story about oranges. Ask parents to send favorite recipes using oranges or orange juice. Decorate the cafeteria with student-made "Orange you glad you eat oranges?" posters. The ideas are endless.

Overkill? Perhaps. But this example illustrates how one nutrition concept — oranges are a tasty and healthful food — can be integrated into the entire school environment. Students pick up skills in science (making orange juice and planting seeds), language arts (writing a story) and art (making posters). Staff, parents and the school cafeteria all become involved, too, making this an integrated effort, the next concept in the F.I.B. approach.

Integrate Nutrition Wherever Possible

Success with nutrition education largely depends on how well it is integrated into other subject areas, intertwined with the school cafeteria and reinforced through food experiences at home.

With barely enough time to teach students core subjects such as math, science and reading, teachers struggle to find time to teach nutrition. It's not that educators aren't interested in nutrition. In a survey of Connecticut teachers, 98 percent of elementary teachers felt that nutrition should be taught in school, but only 56 percent reported teaching nutrition to their students.

In a study published in 2011, researchers in Michigan found that school staff felt that students received too little nutrition education, physical activity, and physical education. Time within the school day and lack of funds were the biggest barriers.

Lack of teacher training is also a barrier to nutrition education. Only about half of teachers have had formal training to teach nutrition, according to a report from the National Center for Education Statistics.

While teachers prefer to integrate nutrition into other subject areas, they don't always have the time or skills to accomplish this goal. Studies show that when nutrition is an integral part of the school day, teachers teach more nutrition over the course of the year than when they present it as a separate unit. You will find dozens of activities and strategies for integrating nutrition into all curricular areas in chapters 4-11.

THE CAFETERIA

Once thought of as a necessary distraction, the school nutrition program is gaining respect as an adjunct to the education of students. As they serve kids breakfast and lunch, nutrition staff who receive proper training can also be enlisted to serve good-nutrition messages.

As school nutrition directors strive to implement kid-accepted menus that meet the new nutrition standards outlined in the Healthy, Hunger-Free Kids Act of 2010, their success will depend on the strength of their integration with the classroom and school community.

To be truly effective, the food and messages received in the school cafeteria should complement nutrition instruction by teachers. A solid nutrition education program in the classroom will confuse and dismay students if they are faced with a display of empty calorie foods in the cafeteria. Likewise, making healthful meal changes without teaching students, parents and school staff the rationale behind the menu switch will likely result in a lot of grumbling and a drop in cafeteria sales.

TAKING THE MESSAGE HOME

It is essential to link school-based nutrition education with the home environment. Through parent meetings, interaction with parent-teacher groups, school events, newsletters, menus, recipes and information sent home, good nutrition concepts can be reinforced. Parents also have a lot to contribute to this effort. Joining their children at school meals, setting up health and nutrition fairs, assisting with classroom nutrition lessons, volunteering in the school kitchen or cafeteria or selling nutritious foods as a fundraiser for education projects are important ways parents can become involved in school nutrition.

Since the bulk of purchasing, food preparation and eating happens at home, kids may need to serve as nutrition teachers, too, encouraging parents to buy and try new foods and experiment with different cooking methods. Assigning cooking "homework" is one way to get the family (and maybe even the dog) involved.

Table 3-1

Effective Nutrition Education: What the Research Shows

According to a report published in the Journal of Nutrition Education, the following components contribute to successful nutrition education with elementary-aged students:

- Instruction with a behavioral focus (better to focus on changing specific behaviors rather than on just learning nutrition facts)
- Use of active learning strategies (not just lectures)
- Devotion of adequate time and intensity to nutrition education (the time needed to impact attitudes and behavior is estimated at 50 hours per year)
- A family involvement component
- School meals and food-related policies that reinforce classroom nutrition education
- Teachers with adequate training in nutrition education

Lytle, L. (1995). Nutrition education for school-aged children. *Journal of Nutrition Education*, 27(6), 298-311.

Emphasize Behavior Change

Nutrition is not just another subject. Like health or physical education, the goal reaches beyond the acquisition of knowledge. Ultimately, we want to produce changes in the daily eating behavior of children. As the example above illustrates, knowing oranges are nutritious isn't enough — eating more oranges is the ultimate goal.

Behavior change does not happen quickly, particularly in adults. It is a process — an evolution that requires a cycle of attempts and failures to finally succeed. That is why some smokers quit and start many times before finally quitting. Or those seeking a healthy weight lose, plateau, gain and lose weight over and over again.

Nutrition Education Essentials

Promote a Healthy Body Image
An overarching theme in working with youngsters of all ages should be to promote a healthy body image and emphasize healthy eating and activity habits. It is important to promote educational practices with children that encourage healthy behaviors as opposed to weight control.

Get Kids Excited about Healthy Eating
When planning nutrition lessons for children, the best approach is to involve kids in activities which are fun, creative and challenging. Children love to contribute to discussions, enjoy hands-on tasks more than lectures, and are especially fond of lessons that involve food preparation and tasting.

Consider Readiness to Learn
Developmental level refers to the level of readiness to learn various concepts and tasks. Just as we wouldn't teach multiplication before a child has mastered addition or attempt reading when we don't know the alphabet, it's important that health and nutrition education start with core concepts and build sequentially.

Teaching nutrition to children early and often is the key to developing healthy eating habits. Fortunately, it is easier to produce nutrition and health behavior change in children. Especially before age 12, children are much more likely to take concepts they learn and put them to practice. In a Minnesota study that tracked children from grade six through adolescence, kids who learned to make positive health decisions in regard to smoking, physical activity and food choices prior to sixth grade ended up with healthier habits as teens. An encouraging follow-up to the CATCH (Child and Adolescent Trial for Cardiovascular Health) Study found that three years after their last formal exposure to vigorous physical activity and nutrition lessons, the eighth graders continued to practice many of the heart-healthy behaviors they had learned in elementary school.

A Philadelphia study published in 2008 found that a multicomponent policy-based school intervention (which included a recommended 50 hours of nutrition instruction) can be effective in preventing obesity among children in grades 4 through 6 in urban public schools.

However, teaching nutrition once a year as a unit, regardless of intensity, will have little impact on long-term behavior change. Those concepts need to be reinforced all year, for many years, to make appreciable changes.

Lessons aimed at behavior change have two things in common: 1) real experience with food and 2) a real-life, reachable goal. Research done with CookShop, a food-based nutrition education program based in New York, showed that when the curriculum included cooking in the classroom, students ate more of the same foods (grains and vegetables) served in the cafeteria.

For instance, a lesson about whole grains might include a whole grain bread baking activity and end by encouraging students to eat at least three servings of whole grains each day. Devising a chart to check off how many whole grains are eaten gives students a chance to sharpen math skills. Homework could consist of a simple whole grain muffin or trail mix recipe for the students to try with their families. The school cafeteria might highlight whole grain foods that week, even including a few new ones such as barley, whole wheat couscous or quinoa. Again, this is an example of an integrated approach to nutrition education aimed at behavior change.

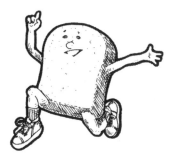

Table 3-2

Nutrition Notes From a Fifth Grade Teacher

In February our class took a good look at our daily eating habits. Each student kept a record of what he or she ate for four days. Students discovered that they had some nutritional holes! Many students were not eating enough grains, vegetables and fruits.

Students set goals to try to eat more food from the food group in which they weren't getting enough servings. They then kept a record of their eating habits for four more days. The results? Most students improved their eating habits. All students became more aware of how many servings per day they should have of each kind of food and what it means to eat a balanced diet.

We learned about how eating a balanced diet can help improve our health, and which foods contain nutrients such as vitamin C, potassium and calcium. We also learned that eating a breakfast made up of foods from at least three food groups can help them do better in school!

A healthful snack of food from at least two food groups can help boost their energy and concentration during the school day. For snack time, students are encouraged to bring healthful snacks, and now, most do. Many of the kids in our classroom are involved in sports or physical play after school. Connie Evers, a registered dietitian (and Sam's mom), came into our classroom to show us how to eat healthfully for athletic activities. We learned that active bodies need carbohydrates to help them stay full of energy. Students also learned that drinking water before, during and after an athletic event is important. Mrs. Evers showed us how to make fruit garnishes out of kiwi and strawberries. Yum!

Students made posters for the cafeteria encouraging other students in our school to eat a well-balanced meal.

Source: Jennifer (Hansen) Butler, Hansen's Headlines, parent newsletter, March 2001.

The Bottom Line

Perhaps the best case for promoting good eating behavior is the immediate effects it has on learning and development. A child who is hungry or poorly nourished is not ready to learn. Nutrition education done right is a boost for education in general. Practicing good nutrition habits makes kids better learners of all subjects.

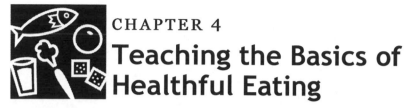

CHAPTER 4

Teaching the Basics of Healthful Eating

"I've been cooking for my family for years, and I've always made well-balanced meals with every food group." —Allison, age 10

Grasping the concept of food groups has long been a goal of nutrition education. While the names, number and emphasis of the food group classification system has changed over the years, the basic principles have remained the same. Simply put, we need to eat different kinds of foods in varying amounts to keep our bodies functioning at full capacity. The three keywords often used to describe the food group system are *variety, balance* and *moderation.*

Nutrition scientists continue to study and discover the most optimal diet that contributes to lifelong health. To reflect this knowledge, the United States Department of Agriculture (USDA) introduced the Dietary Guidelines for Americans (DGA), 2010 (see Dietaryguidelines.gov) and *MyPlate,* the corresponding food guide. The DGA and *MyPlate* recognize that Americans of all ages are increasingly unhealthy and unfit. The *MyPlate*

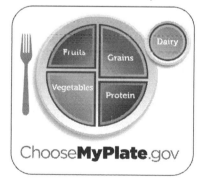

graphic is an easily recognizable symbol which shows a place setting that reflects healthful foods in the proper proportions. The website address is part of the symbol and directs users to choosemyplate.gov for specific advice on food plans and exercise.

The site also includes information for children, including coloring sheets and the *Blast Off Game,* an interactive computer game where kids can reach Planet Power by fueling their rocket with food and physical activity. Other *MyPlate* teaching resources for children can be found at the Team Nutrition website at http://teamnutrition.usda.gov.

Table 4-1

Highlights of MyPlate

▲ AN EASY TO UNDERSTAND GRAPHIC SYMBOL

MyPlate is a graphic presentation of a healthful daily diet. It was designed as an easy tool with all five food groups in the proper amounts, with a key emphasis to **"make half your plate fruits and vegetables."** Everyone from preschoolers to seniors can recognize that *MyPlate* is a place setting with sections for all five food groups.

▲ A COMPREHENSIVE WEBSITE WITH NUTRITION & PHYSICAL ACTIVITY TOOLS

The choosemyplate.gov website provides a wealth of resources on eating healthfully and getting fit. In addition to simplified messages and easy-to-read handouts, there is a comprehensive feature known as **SuperTracker**, which can help you plan, analyze, and track your diet and physical activity.

▲ FOOD GROUP NAMES & MESSAGES

The food group names and messages have been slightly updated:
• Grains — Make at least half your grains whole.
• Vegetables — Vary your veggies.
• Fruits — Focus on fruits.
• Dairy — Get your calcium-rich foods.
• Protein Foods — Go lean with protein.

▲ SERVING SIZES

In an effort to relate more effectively to Americans, servings are listed in U.S. household measurements such as cups and ounces.

▲ EMPHASIS ON WHOLE GRAINS

Because they contain the entire grain kernel, whole grains possess more fiber, vitamins, minerals and phytonutrients than refined grains. A minimum of three servings of whole grains are recommended for most children and adults each day. Examples:
• Bulgur (cracked wheat)   • Brown Rice   • Oatmeal   • Quinoa   • Popcorn
• Stone-ground cornmeal or grits (not the degerminated varieties)
• Grain foods made with 100% whole-grain flour, such as breads, cereals, and pasta
• Cereals made from wheat bran (or that contain added wheat bran)

▲ HEALTHFUL FAT SOURCES

While not a food group, the choosemyplate.gov website includes information on oils and healthful fats. Most nutrition experts agree that there is an advantage to choosing fats such as olive oil, canola oil, avocados, olives, nuts and fatty fish rather than the saturated fats found in animal products, partially hydrogenated fats (also known as trans fats) and saturated vegetable fats such as coconut oil and palm kernel oil. (See more about dietary fat on page 171.)

▲ EMPTY CALORIES*

While the average American consumes 35% of calories from solid fats and added sugars, the recommendation is more in the range of 10-15% for most people, depending on individual age, gender and activity level. (While not a calorie source, sodium, which is found in salt and many processed foods, should also be limited.)

*NOTE: To simplify this concept for children, this category will be referred to in this book as "extra" foods. Most children who eat a balanced diet can fit in 1-2 servings of "extra" foods each day. The trick, however, is to exercise portion control and to read and understand Nutrition Facts labels. Chips, candy, soft drinks, cookies and other "extras" often contain several servings in one package.

HOW MUCH?

Table 4-2 provides information on the food groups, how much is needed each day and examples of foods in each food group. To obtain a personalized *Daily Food Plan*, visit choosemyplate.gov.

Teaching MyPlate

Before you begin your basic nutrition unit, be sure to obtain a classroom-sized *MyPlate* poster for reference from the Team Nutrition website located at http://teamnutrition.usda.gov. You can also use a classroom projector to show images of *MyPlate*, food groups and other resources located at choosemyplate.gov. The mini-poster *What's on Your Plate* is located at http://www.choosemyplate.gov/downloads/mini_poster_English_final.pdf .

CONCEPTS TO TEACH

The following points outline the key messages children should ultimately grasp when studying *MyPlate*.

▲ There are five different food groups represented in the *MyPlate* graphic. The space taken up on the plate and accompanying blue circle (or glass) represents the approximate proportion of that food group in the diet.

▲ Each food group provides a unique set of nutrients that helps our body perform at full capacity. The body needs a total of about 40 nutrients, which fall into six general classes: **Carbohydrates**, **Protein**, **Fat**, **Vitamins**, **Minerals** and **Water**. Eating foods from all the food groups is the best way to get the nutrients needed for good health (see Table 4-3).

In addition to the basic nutrients, there are also a whole host of functional compounds found in many foods that benefit the body in a variety of ways. Plant-based foods such as fruits, vegetables, grains, beans, nuts and seeds contain hundreds of "phytonutrients," which are non-nutrient plant compounds thought to protect body cells and prevent chronic disease. Foods with beneficial chemicals are also known as "functional foods." Table 4-4 provides some examples of specific functional compounds found in a variety of food and beverages.

Table 4-2

MyPlate: Recommended Servings for Children ages 6-11*			
FOOD GROUP	**AMOUNT NEEDED EACH DAY**	**EXAMPLES**	**GO EASY ON**
Grains	5 to 7 ounces (at least half from whole grain sources)	1 ounce is approximately: 1 slice of bread; 1 cup of dry cereal; ½ cup of rice, pasta, or cooked cereal; 3 cups of popcorn; 1 small tortilla; 7 round crackers	Refined grains and grains with added sugars
Vegetables	1 ½ to 2 ½ cups	1 cup cooked or chopped vegetables; 2 cups salad greens is considered 1 cup from the vegetable group. Emphasize deep orange, dark green, red, purple and other colorful vegetables.	High fat salad dressings, butter added to cooked vegetables, and fried vegetables such as French fries
Fruits	1 ½ cups to 2 cups	1 cup of fruit or 100% juice; Also equal to 1 cup of fruit: 1 small apple; 1 large banana; 1 large orange; 32 grapes; ½ cup dried fruit	Fruit with added sugar Limit fruit juice to 4-8 oz. daily.
Dairy	2 ½ cups (ages 4 to 8) 3 cups (age 9 and older)	1 cup of milk or yogurt or 1½ ounces of cheese; 8 oz. of calcium-fortified soy beverage (soymilk)	High fat cheeses and high sugar dairy desserts
Protein Foods	4 to 6 ounces total of meat or meat equivalents	1 ounce lean meat, poultry, or seafood; ¼ cup beans, 1 egg, 1 Tablespoon of peanut butter, ½ ounce (about 2 Tablespoons) of shelled sunflower seeds or nuts	High fat and/or cured meats, poultry with the skin left on, and fried protein foods
Limit "Extra" foods such as candy, chocolate, cookies, donuts, sweetened drinks, and fried chips to no more than 1 to 2 servings on most days.			

*For a personalized *Daily Food Plan* based on your age, gender, height, weight and activity level, visit www.choosemyplate.gov.

▲ The fruit and vegetable groups are important because they provide a whole host of vitamins, minerals, carbohydrates, fiber and phytonutrients. Half of our daily food volume should come from fruits and vegetables. Children need approximately 1½ to 2 cups of fruit and 1½ to 2½ cups of vegetables each day for good health, a strong immune system, and a healthy appearance. The nutrients found in fruits and vegetables are important for keeping our skin, eyes and hair healthy. Vibrant colors are an indication that produce is rich in nutrients as well as functional components. Include vegetables and fruits that are dark green, deep yellow/orange, red, blue, and purple.

Beans are a Super Food
Dry beans, split peas and lentils are rich in protein and also provide fiber, potassium, iron, folate, magnesium and many other nutrients. Because of their unique composition, they can be counted as either a vegetable or protein serving.

▲ Grains are rich in energy-giving carbohydrates, B vitamins, iron and fiber. Our bodies' first and most important need is for energy. Besides the energy it takes for movement, play and sports, we also use energy just to stay alive. With each breath, heartbeat or blink of the eyes, we are expending energy.

The average child needs a total of about 5 to 7 ounces of grains daily, with at least half coming from whole grains. Whole grains possess more fiber, vitamins, minerals and phytonutrients than refined grains, which have had the outer covering (bran) and germ removed. Regular consumption of whole grains is important for digestive health, reduces the rate of coronary heart disease and decreases the risk of several types of cancer. Surveys show that most Americans of all ages are lucky to consume even one daily serving of whole grains.

Fiber, while not a nutrient in the true sense, helps the body to move food through the digestive system. Fiber also helps our health in other ways, too (e.g., some fibers lower blood cholesterol and stabilize blood sugar levels). Whole grains such as brown rice and 100 percent whole-wheat bread have more fiber than refined white rice or bread made from enriched flour. Other fiber-rich foods include beans, fruits and vegetables.

Table 4-3

Nutrients and What They Do		
FOOD GROUP	**KEY NUTRIENTS***	**ACTION IN THE BODY**
Grains	Carbohydrate, Fiber, B vitamins, Iron	**Carbohydrate** is the body's major source of energy. **Fiber** aids the movement of food through the digestive tract. **B vitamins** help in the body's use of energy. **Iron** carries oxygen in red blood cells and muscle cells.
Vegetables	Vitamin A, Vitamin C, Folate, Iron, Magnesium, Fiber	**Vitamin A** helps maintain skin and mucous membranes and aids in vision. **Vitamin C** helps the body heal and fight infections. **Folate** is needed for healthy blood cells and is important for cell division, such as in pregnancy and growth. **Magnesium** is found in bones and is important for muscle and nerve functioning.
Fruits	Vitamin A, Vitamin C, Potassium, Folate, Fiber	**Potassium** maintains the heart beat, regulates body fluids, and is needed for muscle and nerve functioning.
Dairy	Calcium, Vitamin D, Potassium, Protein Riboflavin	**Calcium** is needed for the development and maintenance of healthy bones and teeth. **Vitamin D** is needed for bone health and immune function. **Riboflavin** is a B vitamin that helps the body use energy.
Protein Foods	Protein, B vitamins, Iron, Zinc	**Protein** provides the building blocks needed for growth, replacement and maintenance of body tissues. **Zinc** is necessary for healing, taste perception, growth and sexual development.
Oils (not a food group)	Essential fatty acids	**Essential Fatty Acids** are needed for brain development and function, healthy cell membranes and normal growth and development.
Empty Calories (not a food group)	Simple Carbohydrates (sugars), Solid Fats	**Simple carbohydrates** or sugars provide energy but few other nutrients. **Solid Fats** such as animal fats, artificial trans fats (partially hydrogenated vegetable oils) and tropical oils may increase the risk of heart disease.

*There are more than 40 different nutrients with many different functions that are required for good health. Each food group contributes many other nutrients in addition to the "key nutrients" listed here.

Table 4-4

Foods with Functional Components

While we have long understood that food provides essential nutrients, nutrition experts now realize that hundreds of non-nutrient phytonutrients and other compounds may promote optimal health, protect body cells and lower the risk of chronic diseases such as cancer and cardiovascular disease.

Scientists are only beginning to unravel the questions of how functional components work or how much is needed to exert a protective effect. By including a wide variety of whole, unprocessed foods in your daily diet, you will automatically consume many protective substances. Below are a few examples.

FUNCTIONAL COMPONENT	POSSIBLE HEALTH BENEFITS	FOOD SOURCES
Anthocyanins	Antioxidant that may protect against effects of aging	Blueberries, plums, cherries, strawberries
Beta Glucan (soluble fiber)	Lowers blood cholesterol levels	Oats
Catechins	Reduces the risk of cancer	Black and green tea
Elagic Acid	Reduces the risk of cancer; Lowers blood cholesterol levels	Red grapes, kiwifruit, blueberries, raspberries, strawberries, blackberries
Lutein	Promotes eye health (especially as we age)	Dark green leafy vegetables, kiwifruit, broccoli
Lycopene	Reduces the risk of prostate cancer and heart disease	Tomatoes, red pepper, pink grapefruit, watermelon
Omega-3 Fatty acids	Reduces the risk for heart disease; Plays a role in joint, eye, and brain health.	Cold-water fish such as salmon, mackerel, herring and sardines; Flaxseed oil, walnuts
Probiotics	Aids gastrointestinal health	Yogurt and other fermented dairy products
Sulforaphane	Reduces the risk of cancer	Broccoli, cauliflower, cabbage, Brussels sprouts
Sulfur Compounds	Reduces the risk of cancer; Lowers blood cholesterol and blood pressure	Garlic, onions, chives, leeks, scallions

For more information on functional foods, visit:
http://www.foodinsight.org/Resources/Detail.aspx?topic=Background_on_functional_Foods

▲ Dairy foods provide a nutrient-rich package with key levels of calcium, protein, vitamins A, D, and B12, riboflavin, niacin, potassium and phosphorus. Kids ages 9 and older need 3 servings of dairy each day, while children 4 to 8 years old need 2½ servings, and children 2 to 3 years old need 2 servings. A serving of dairy is 8 ounces or 1 cup of yogurt or milk and 1½ ounces of cheese. To cut down on saturated fat, a switch to fat-free or low-fat milk is recommended for adults and children ages 2 and up. Fat-free and low-fat milk have the same key nutrients as whole milk, but fewer calories and fat.

▲ The protein foods group is rich in many nutrients, including protein, B vitamins, iron and zinc. Protein is vital because it contains the building blocks for growth, development and repair. Most children require around 4 to 6 ounces of meat or meat equivalents each day. To maximize nutrition, choose seafood, lean meats, poultry without the skin, beans, nuts and seeds. The 2010 DGA and *MyPlate* recommend that seafood should be the protein on your plate twice each week.

> **What if milk poses a problem for you?**
>
> ♦ For those who are lactose intolerant, smaller portions (such as 2 to 4 fluid ounces of milk) may be tolerated. Lactose-free and lower-lactose products are also available and enzyme preparations can be added to milk to lower the lactose content.
>
> ♦ Aged cheeses such as cheddar, Monterey Jack and Swiss are naturally low in lactose. Cultured dairy foods such as yogurt are typically well tolerated because they contain friendly bacteria that help digest lactose.
>
> ♦ If you follow a vegetarian diet that includes no animal products (known as a vegan) or have a milk allergy, you need to include non-dairy sources of calcium in your diet such as a calcium-fortified soy beverage, calcium-set tofu, calcium-fortified fruit juices, broccoli, kale, almonds and calcium-fortified breakfast cereals.
>
> ♦ If you eat fish, calcium-rich sources include sardines and canned salmon (canned with the bones).

KNOWING HOW MUCH TO EAT

Most kids need to eat at least the minimum amount recommended from each food group. But many kids will need more, especially those who are active in movement, sports and play. Here is one way to explain this to children:

> "How much you eat is entirely up to you. Well, at least it's up to your body. While dietitians can use complicated equations to figure out about how many calories you need for growth, activity and energy, they can also be

wrong. That is because your body is a one-of-a-kind. You are growing and changing and your activity level is not always the same. Some days you need more calories and some days you need fewer.

The best way to know how much to eat is to listen to your body! Eat only when you are hungry (not bored or sad or frustrated) and only until your body feels comfortably full.

A rating scale like the one below can help you to learn how much to eat. It's best to eat when your stomach feels about like a "2" on the chart below and stop eating at "3." When you wait to eat until you are at "1," you may want to eat everything in sight. When you keep eating until "4" or "5," you can end up putting too much energy in your body, which will be stored as extra fat. The best way to know how much to eat is to listen to your body! Eat until your body feels comfortably full. You should feel satisfied but not overly stuffed."

ACTIVITY

HOW FULL ARE YOU?

Lead children in a discussion of how it feels to eat too much, not enough and just the right amount. Next, ask them to develop a rating scale for hunger and fullness, with 1 being really hungry and 5 being overstuffed (like Thanksgiving).

Example:

Starving!	My stomach feels empty.	I feel just right - not too hungry or too full.	I'm feeling too full.	I ate way too much! I don't feel so well.
1	2	3	4	5

For 1–3 days, ask the children to use the scale to note their level of hunger/fullness before and after each meal. Ask them if they noticed any patterns. Are they eating about the right amount of food? Discuss how this assignment can help them to regulate their food to more closely match their bodies' needs.

AVOIDING MyPlate OVERLOAD

Break *MyPlate* concepts into several sessions so children can fully "digest" the material. Each session should ideally have a hands-on, discovery activity (see next section for ideas). Below is a suggested timeline for presenting information, although it will vary according to age and developmental level.

▲Session 1: Introduce the *MyPlate* graphic and explain how foods for good health are divided into five main food groups. Plan activities that allow students to sort and categorize foods into the five food groups. (For active games that teach students the five food groups, see the **Food Games** section, starting on page 180.) Discuss how each section on the *MyPlate* graphic is a different size, which means we need more servings from the groups with the bigger sections.

▲Session 2: Review the serving amounts suggested for each food group. Lead students in a discussion of "How much food do I need?" Set up measuring centers where students can discover the serving sizes of various foods.

▲Session 3: Introduce the concept of nutrients and list the six classes (Carbohydrates, Protein, Fat, Vitamins, Minerals, Water). Explain that because each food group contains a different set of nutrients, we need foods from all the groups to get the nutrients our bodies need. Highlight how key nutrients are needed to build and maintain a healthy body (see Table 4-3). Discuss with older students the concept of the beneficial chemicals in food known as functional components. (see Table 4-4).

▲Session 4: Ask the class for examples of empty calorie "extra" foods that do not fit into any of the *MyPlate* groups. Discuss the concept of dietary excess (e.g., how we need to limit foods that are high in sugar, fat and sodium) and the importance of eating these foods in moderation (i.e., limiting to no more than 1-2 servings on most days).

Planning MyPlate Activities

To bring alive the concepts of *MyPlate*, plan activities that will engage students and make the food groups relevant to their lives.

ACTIVITIES

▲ 15 USES FOR A BLANK MYPLATE

The blank *MyPlate* on page 52 can be used in a variety of ways to teach *MyPlate* concepts. Photocopy or scan page 52 or download one of the original blank coloring sheets from the children's section of choosemyplate.gov. Assign children the following activities or create your own.

1. Display a colored poster or projected graphic of *MyPlate*. Pass out blank *MyPlate* sheets and ask children to color and label the sections with the food group names. As time allows, they can also draw pictures of foods from each food group.

> **Evaluation Tip:** *You can also do this activity as a pre-test before showing children the poster in order to assess whether they can correctly identify the food groups and their position on the MyPlate guide. Upon completion of your nutrition unit, repeat this exercise to see if they can easily identify all groups in the proper spaces.*

2. Bring in gardening catalogs, food magazines and/or weekly food advertisements from the newspaper. Ask students to cut out the pictures and paste on the blank *MyPlate* in the appropriate food group sections. You can also set this up as a self-directed center in a designated classroom area.

3. Use a blank *MyPlate* as a daily diet record. Carry it with you and record each food you eat or drink in the appropriate food group section. Break foods into their components (e.g., record a soup made of noodles, beef and vegetables in the grains, protein and vegetable groups). Check your record for balance. Is there a lot of blank space in certain groups? Are other groups overcrowded? Are there changes you could make to better balance your *MyPlate*?

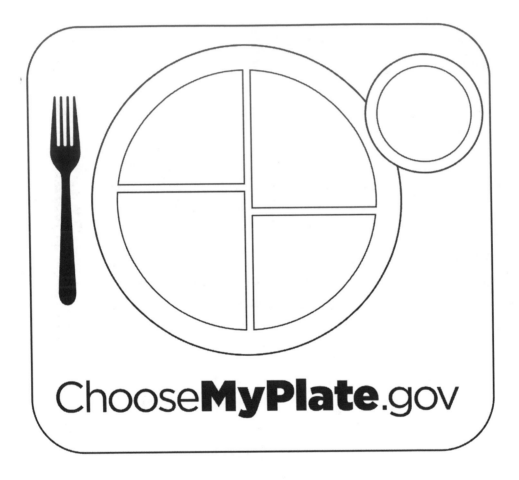

ChooseMyPlate.gov

For additional options for blank *MyPlate* sheets, visit the kids section at http://www.choosemyplate.gov/children-over-five.html.

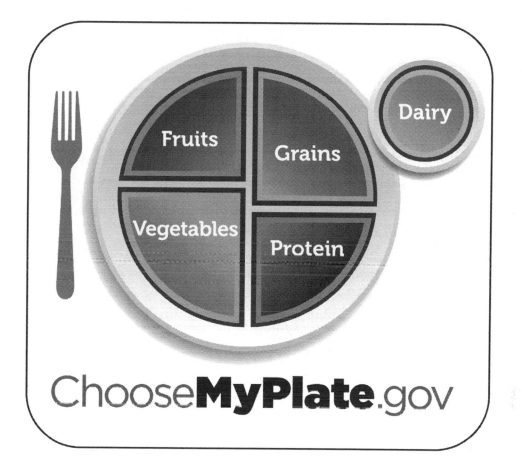

ChooseMyPlate.gov

4. Chart today's school breakfast and/or lunch menus on the blank *MyPlate*. Are the menus balanced? Would you make any changes to the meals?

5. Ask the children who brought a packed lunch from home to take a look at how the foods in their lunch fit on the blank *MyPlate*. Are most of the food groups represented? Would you make any changes to the meal?

6. Use *MyPlate* to plan your after-school or bedtime snack. Close your eyes and think about what foods are usually available in your refrigerator, freezer, pantry or cupboard. Next, think about which of these foods would make a good *MyPlate* snack. Write down or draw this snack on the blank *MyPlate*. Try to include at least two to three different food groups in your snack.

7. Plan a *MyPlate* meal that you can cook yourself. It can be as simple as a sandwich of peanut butter with sliced fruit on whole grain bread with 1% milk or as complicated as a seafood stir-fry over brown rice with 1% milk and fruit salad. Remember, you are the cook.

8. Draw a vegetarian *MyPlate*. What foods would you include in the protein group? What about the dairy group? Do vegetarians eat eggs? (ANSWER: Vegetarian diets are varied. Some, called lacto-vegetarians, include milk, yogurt and cheese in their diets. Lacto-ovo-vegetarians also eat eggs. Strict vegetarians, known as vegans, eat only plant-based foods and often include foods such as calcium-fortified soy milk and tofu in their diets.)

9. Draw an ethnic *MyPlate*. Pick a culture that you are studying about or interested in and research what types of foods are commonly eaten by the people of that culture. For example, a Mexican *MyPlate* might include tortillas (grains), beans (protein), cheese (dairy) and salsa (vegetables). What would a Middle Eastern, Chinese or Italian *MyPlate* look like?

10. Many of the foods commonly eaten by Americans are mixed dishes comprised of several ingredients. Sandwiches, soups and stews, stir-fry dishes, lasagna, tacos, pizza, and smoothies are all examples of combination foods. To make sense of the nutrition of mixed foods, a little dissection is in order. You first need to separate the foods you eat into their individual parts. Using the blank *MyPlate*, write the components in the proper food group sections. Use one of the following examples or create your own:

VEGETARIAN PIZZA: whole-wheat crust, tomato sauce with spices, part-skim mozzarella cheese, red pepper rings, mushrooms, onions, black olives

CHINESE STIR-FRY: water chestnuts, bean sprouts, pea pods, broccoli florets, chicken pieces, peanuts, brown rice

SUB SANDWICH: Whole-wheat hoagie roll, sliced turkey, lean ham, part-skim mozzarella cheese, tomato slices, shredded lettuce, pickle slices, oil, vinegar

11. Research the foods that are grown in your state or region. Design a "*MyPlate* where I live," filling in all of the local agricultural products in the correct food group sections. A good place to find facts on agriculture for all 50 states is at the USDA Agriculture in the Classroom website located at http://agclassroom.org/kids/ag_facts.htm. Another source for information on locally grown foods is http://www.localharvest.org.

12. Research the nutrients that each food group provides. Write the key nutrients from each group on the proper section of the blank *MyPlate*. (ANSWERS: Grains — carbohydrate, fiber, B vitamins, iron; Vegetables — vitamins A and C, folate, iron, magnesium, fiber; Fruits — vitamins A and C, potassium, folate, fiber; Dairy — calcium, vitamin D, riboflavin, potassium, protein; Protein — protein, B vitamins, iron, zinc.) Refer to Table 4-3 on page 46 for more about specific nutrients.

13. Draw a "body-part" *MyPlate* that represents how each food group helps different parts of the body. EXAMPLE: Draw an exercising body in the grain space, healthy eyes in the vegetable group, glowing hair and skin for the fruit group, an arm posing a muscle in the protein group and a healthy, toothy smile for the dairy group.

14. Make a giant *MyPlate* to decorate the school cafeteria. Start with a large blank *MyPlate*. Assign seven students to the grains group, five to the vegetables group, three to the fruits group, three to the dairy group and three to the protein group (you may need to make adjustments according to class size). Have students design, draw, paint, sculpt or color a

favorite food from their assigned food group. Paste the food pictures or sculptures on the large *MyPlate* and hang or display it in the cafeteria. Be sure to have students sign their artwork. Another idea is to enlist the help of an artist or art teacher and have the students design and paint a *MyPlate* mural directly onto the cafeteria wall.

15. HOMEWORK: Accompany the "family shopper" on the next trip to the grocery store. Are most foods in the store from one of the five food groups? As the groceries are being put away at home, write down all the items on your blank *MyPlate* record. Is your *MyPlate* balanced? What suggestions would you give the family shopper (nicely, of course)?

⊞ MAKE A FOOD GROUP COUNTER

Using a shoe box, string or twine and buttons or beads, children can create an abacus-like device to help them count how many food group servings they eat each day. First, punch six small holes along one of the long sides of the shoebox. Punch six more on the other side that pair up with the first set of holes. Next, cut six pieces of string that are approximately twice the width of the box. Knot each piece of string and thread through the holes. Feed 12 beads or buttons onto each string. The last step is to thread the string through the opposite hole and tie a knot on the end to secure.

You Will Need:

For each Food Group Counter:

♦ Shoebox

♦ string or twine

♦ 72 buttons or beads (evenly divided among six different colors)

♦ markers or crayons

Each row of beads represents a food group. Match the bead/button colors to the groups if possible: grains:orange, vegetables:green, fruits:red, dairy:blue, protein:purple, and a separate color for "extra foods." NOTE: It is easier to write the food group names on the bottom of the box before stringing the beads.

Ask students to record the foods they eat each day. (The *MyPlate* diet record suggested in #3 on page 51 above works well.) Using their Food Group Counter, the students can move one bead to the opposite side for each serving they eat in that category. They can also do this for individual meals, snacks or school meal menus. This

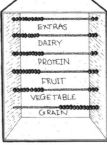

device will give students a visual tool that allows them to immediately gauge whether a meal or diet is balanced.

MEASURING CENTERS

Perhaps the biggest hang-up in applying *MyPlate* to daily eating habits is confusion over serving sizes (this is true of adults as well as children). Hands-on experience weighing and measuring different foods will give children a better grasp of what a so-called "serving" looks like.

Set up centers for children to manipulate and measure real food. Small food scales, measuring cups, measuring spoons, plates, cups and bowls are needed for this activity.

CAUTION: This is *not* an eating activity, since everyone will be touching the food. You may want to plan this activity in conjunction with a snack or conduct it right after lunch, when tummies are full.

Some suggestions for centers:

• Measure 1 ounce (1/2 cup) of cooked spaghetti, noodles, macaroni or rice onto a dinner-sized plate.

• Weigh 1½ ounces of cheese in different forms, including sliced, cubed or grated.

• Measure one teaspoon of soft trans-fat bread spread/margarine or slice one "pat" of stick butter (using lines on butter wrapper).

• Pour 1 cup of 100 percent fruit juice into a glass.

• Using whole leaves from leaf lettuce or fresh spinach, tear into bite-sized pieces and measure 2 cups. How many lettuce leaves does it take to fill 2 cups?

• Weigh 1 ounce of drained, canned tuna fish.

• Set up a "guess table" with a variety of foods. The objective is to guess how many servings each food item really provides. Examples include an English muffin (2 ounces of

You Will Need:
♦ Measuring cups
♦ Measuring spoons
♦ Food scale
♦ Serving utensils
♦ Plates, cups and bowls
♦ Cooked pasta or rice
♦ Cheese
♦ Butter or trans-fat free spread
♦ Fruit juice
♦ Salad greens
♦ Tuna fish
♦ Items for "guess table" (see text)

grains), 1 cup canned fruit, 1 large orange (1 serving), 32 grapes, 1 cup cooked oatmeal (2 ounces grains), 1/2 pint carton of milk (1 cup), 1/2 ounce shelled sunflower seeds (1 ounce meat equivalent) or a 3-ounce cooked hamburger patty (3 ounces of protein).

Your school cafeteria manager is the real expert when it comes to serving sizes. Part of the manager's job is to make sure that cafeteria staff is serving the right-sized portions. Invite him/her into the classroom to demonstrate different scoops, scales and spoons used to control serving sizes. Also encourage students to take note of the serving sizes on their school breakfast and lunch trays. For instance, a typical pre-plated school lunch has 2 ounces of meat or protein, 1 cup of milk, 1–2 ounces of grains and approximately ½ cup fruits and 1 cup of vegetables.

USING MYPLATE IN DRAMATIC PLAY AREAS

Setting up dramatic play areas is a great way for primary students (K-third grade) to play and practice the concepts of the *MyPlate*.

▲ *MyPlate* Supermarket: Set up a supermarket that is full of *MyPlate* choices. Include shelves for food, grocery carts, aprons, cash register and grocery bags. Decorate the walls with student-made posters and advertisements.

You Will Need:
◆ Shelves
◆ A variety of empty food packages and/or food models
◆ Grocery flyers from the newspaper
◆ Grocery carts
◆ Aprons
◆ Cash register
◆ Grocery sacks (preferably cloth reusable bags)

For food models, use actual food packages such as beans, pasta, quinoa and brown rice; empty oatmeal containers and cereal boxes; milk and yogurt cartons; and stuffed whole grain bread wrappers. For colorful fruit and vegetable models, cut out photos from gardening catalogs and grocery flyers and glue onto foam core. Use rubber models of perishable items such as meat, poultry, seafood and eggs. Include a wide variety of foods from all five food groups and a few foods from the "extras" category.

▲ *MyPlate* Kitchen: Stock the dramatic play area kitchen with healthful *MyPlate* choices. Include real packages or models of low-fat or fat-free milk, yogurt and cheese; lean meats, chicken and seafood; whole grains, including 100 percent whole-wheat bread and flour and plenty of examples of grains, beans, fruits and vegetables.

▲ The *MyPlate* Cafe: Use glasses, plates, silverware, napkins and food pictures that students can make into meals. The food pictures can be preprinted, cut from magazines or food advertisements or made by students. Provide tables and chairs, student-created menus, aprons, chef hats, pads and pencils, a cash register and anything else that your young restaurateurs need to run their cafe.

▲ *MyPlate* Felt Board: Design a *MyPlate* felt board in the shape of the *MyPlate* with a variety of felt foods. (Encourage children to help you design and cut out the foods.) You can also feature a felt placemat with plate, dinnerware, glasses and napkins.

▲ A MyPlate PARTY: CREATE YOUR OWN SANDWICH

A great cooking/tasting activity is to give children an opportunity to create *MyPlate* sandwiches. Check with your cafeteria manager as a source for low-cost food supplies. If eaten as part of a reimbursable school meal, the food items will count as meal components. Funds for nutrition education projects may also be available from the local parent-teacher organization or through nutrition education grants.

NOTE: It is best to conduct this activity as part of lunch or at the end of the school day to avoid interfering with the school meal program.

Beforehand, review Appendix A, "Guidelines for Safe Classroom Cooking." Make sure you communicate with parents and inquire about any food allergies, intolerances or medical conditions that will influence the foods that you can offer. Be sure to enlist parent volunteers to help with this project.

You Will Need:
♦ Plenty of volunteers!
♦ Variety of food items from each food group (see text for ideas)
♦ Serving utensils
♦ Long table
♦ Plastic or latex gloves
♦ Plates
♦ Plastic knives
♦ Napkins

To create *MyPlate* sandwiches, make available a variety of items that can be combined into a large number of sandwich combinations. Try to have at least three choices from each food group available. Below are examples from each food category.

Grains: whole grain bread, rye bread, whole grain flatbread, whole grain bagels, whole corn tortillas, whole grain English muffins, whole-wheat pita bread, whole grain hoagie rolls

Vegetables: lettuce, dark leafy greens such as spinach, arugula or kale leaves, tomato slices, cucumber slices, pepper rings, onion slices, mushroom slices, grated carrots, sliced summer squash, radish slices

Fruits: avocado chunks or slices, banana slices, raisins, applesauce, pineapple tidbits, blueberries, kiwifruit slices

Dairy: low-fat ricotta cheese, low-fat cheese slices, low-fat grated cheese

Protein: peanut, almond or other nut butters; lean sliced turkey, ham or roast beef; water-packed tuna; vegetarian refried beans; hummus

Extras: butter, trans-fat free bread spread/margarine, mayonnaise, jam, jelly

Before you begin, list all of the available food items on the board. Explain to the students that they will get a chance to build their own *MyPlate* sandwich, using any combination of foods they wish. Encourage them to start thinking about the sandwich they wish to make — otherwise the line may move at a snail's pace!

Reading about Eating
Two amusing books to read in conjunction with this activity include *What's Cooking, Jenny Archer?* by Ellen Conford and *Carla's Sandwich* by Debbie Herman.

On a long table, set out all items and arrange by food group. You will also need plastic gloves, plates, plastic knives for spreading and napkins. After thorough handwashing, let small groups of children come to the table. Instruct them to put on plastic gloves and refrain from touching their hair, face, clothing or neighbor.

Encourage students to experiment with new food combinations, building a sandwich that has at least three of the five food groups. After everyone has created a *MyPlate* sandwich, it's time to eat the results!

FOLLOW-UP ACTIVITIES

1. Encourage students to write about their sandwich, including what they liked about it, how they would change it next time, how many food groups they used and whether they think their families or friends would eat it.

2. Ask students to write a fictional story inspired by this activity or the *MyPlate* food guide.

3. The food lists recorded on the board can also be used:
    – To create additional sandwich combinations on paper that the children could try at home.
    – To construct sentences or a story, using as many of the food words as possible.
    – As weekly spelling words.

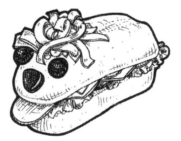

To make this sandwich, see page 159.

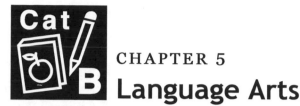

CHAPTER 5

Language Arts

"I really liked your lesson because we got to eat it." —Naveid

Children can explore a variety of nutrition concepts through the language arts. The study and understanding of food and nutrition can be effectively integrated into reading, writing, storytelling, and spelling activities.

Daily Menu Reading

As you change the calendar and discuss the weather each day, consider another daily task — read and discuss the school lunch menu and/or the following day's breakfast menu.

Assign a student to read the menu to the class. As time allows, lead a class discussion about the menu, asking some or all of the following questions.

▲ Can you categorize each menu item according to its food group category? How many different food groups does the menu contain? Does the menu fit the guidelines of *MyPlate*? If there are a variety of food choices offered (e.g. cereal bar or salad bar), is it easy to put together a breakfast or lunch that is nutritious and balanced? Are there any food choices that would be classified as "extra" foods?

▲ Poll students to find out how many will eat the school meal. How many brought their lunch from home?

▲ Ask children what they like the most and least about the menu and to explain their answers. Encourage them to fill in the blank, "If I were the cafeteria manager, I would serve _____."

Predict how many students school-wide will eat either school breakfast or lunch today. How can they find out the answer to their prediction? (HINT: Ask the cafeteria manager.)

Children's Books with Food Themes

Children's literature is full of books with food and nutrition messages. This section highlights a few recommended books and corresponding hands-on activities. The box at left features trusted sources for locating additional books that will match your subject and unit themes.

Sources for Children's Food & Nutrition Books

Neat Solutions for Healthy Children
http://www.neatsolutions.com

Michigan Team Nutrition Booklist
An annotated list of over 400 books with positive food, nutrition and activity messages for children in grades K-2
http://1.usa.gov/wTvW5H

California Ag in the Classroom
The CFAITC website features an extensive list of searchable books related to food, nutrition and agriculture.
http://www.cfaitc.org/books/

The titles selected for this chapter will stimulate discussion, serve as a prelude to a nutrition or cooking activity and promote positive food behaviors.

Before you conduct any of the food activities recommended in this chapter, review Appendix A, "Guidelines for Safe Classroom Cooking." Make sure you communicate with parents and inquire about any food allergies, intolerances or medical conditions that will influence the foods that you can offer.

EARLY ELEMENTARY (K-SECOND GRADES)

♦ **Bread and Jam for Frances**

Hoban, R. & Hoban, L. (2008). *Bread and Jam for Frances*. London: HarperCollins. (reissued edition)

This book is a perfect antidote for children who make limited food choices. Frances's food jag is short-lived once her parents begin serving her bread and jam for every meal and snack. In the end, she agrees with her friend Albert, who declares, "I think it's nice that there are all different kinds of lunches and breakfasts and dinners and snacks. I think eating is nice."

ACTIVITY

▲ Lead a discussion on how choosing a variety of different foods can make eating fun. Encourage children to draw pictures of two or more different breakfasts, lunches or dinners (with no repeating of foods) that they enjoy eating.

◆ **Blueberries for Sal**

Mccloskey, R. (2010). *Blueberries for Sal.* London: Puffin. (reissued edition)

Little Sal gets so involved picking (and eating) blueberries on Blueberry Hill that she loses her mother. Meanwhile, a baby bear cub does the same — and soon the baby bear and Little Sal have swapped moms!

ACTIVITIES

▲ Sample and rate a variety of berries, including blueberries, strawberries and raspberries.

▲ Research or discuss how blueberries and other berries grow.

▲ In late Spring/early Summer, take a field trip to a berry farm.

You Will Need:

◆ Different berries for tasting

◆ Serving bowls and utensils

◆ Small plates

◆ Clean hands

◆ Plastic gloves

◆ **Eating the Alphabet: Fruits & Vegetables from A to Z**

Ehlert, L. (1993). *Eating the Alphabet.* San Diego: Voyager Books.

With beautiful watercolor illustrations, the art in this book will appeal to readers of all ages. The author includes well-known produce with the more exotic, including endive, jicama, kumquat, kohlrabi, quince, ugli fruit and xigua (Chinese watermelon). A highlight of the book is the glossary, which gives descriptions, origins and interesting facts about all of the fruits and vegetables in the book.

ACTIVITIES

▲ Bring in a variety of the fruits and vegetables from Eating the Alphabet to observe and taste.

▲ Take a walking field trip to a grocery market. Tour the produce section, noting the variety of produce available. Write about it later.

▨ Encourage students to create and illustrate their own "Eating the Alphabet" books, using foods from all of the food groups.

▨ ▨ Assign each student a letter of the alphabet. Distribute brown paper bags and assorted art supplies, instruct-

You Will Need:

◆ A variety of fruits and vegetables

◆ Cutting board and knife

◆ Serving bowls and utensils

◆ Small plates

◆ Clean hands

◆ Plastic gloves

ing students to make a puppet that represents a food of that letter. Use the puppets to create a skit or act out "The Alphabet Song."

◆ Green Eggs and Ham

Seuss, D. (1960). *Green eggs and ham*. New York: Random House, Inc. Tongue-tied teachers and parents can take refuge in the fact that Green Eggs and Ham does make an important point about food, i.e. you will never know if you like a new food until you try it. That now-classic refrain is as pertinent today as ever: "You do not like them. So you say. Try them! Try them! And you may. Try them and you may, I say."

ACTIVITIES

▲ Lead a discussion with the children about trying new foods. Ask questions such as: Have you ever decided whether you liked a food before you tasted it? Have you ever been surprised by the taste of a new food? Have you ever set a good example for others by trying new foods?

▲ Have children think of foods that they are hesitant to try, either at home or at school. Award "Sam-I-Am" points each time a child tries any new food of their choice. Reward students with small incentives or privileges after they attain a certain number of points.

◆ Gregory the Terrible Eater

Sharmat, M. (2009). *Gregory, the terrible eater*. New York: Scholastic. This book is a classic tale about the struggles parents and "kids" have over food choices. Gregory the goat refuses the usual goat fare of shoes, old neckties and tin cans in favor of fruits, vegetables, eggs and orange juice.

ACTIVITIES

▲ There are many different nutritious foods from which to choose. Ask children whether it is OK to like some foods better than others. Is it possible to have different food preferences than other family members?

▲ Point out that this is a silly, funny story. While goats do sometimes nibble on paper and clothing, those are not the foods real goats subsist on. Ask children if they have ideas about what goats really do eat. (AN-SWER: hay, alfalfa, oats, corn and apples.)

[Y] Have students design finger and stick puppets of Gregory, his parents, Doctor Ram, foods and other objects from *Gregory the Terrible Eater* and act out the book as a puppet show.

◆ Handa's Surprise

Browne, E. (2011). *Handa's surprise*. Cambridge, Mass: Candlewick Press.

This is a delightful tale of a young Kenyan girl on her way to visit her friend in a nearby village. On the way, seven different animals eat the seven varieties of fruit on her head. Children love seeing the beautiful and colorful illustrations and delight in the surprise twist at the end of the story.

ACTIVITY

▲ Make a classroom fruit salad using some or all of the fruits featured in *Handa's Surprise* (bananas, guavas, oranges, mangos, pineapple, avocado, passion fruit and tangerines). Be sure to show students the whole forms of the fruit before peeling and slicing.

You Will Need:

- Some or all of the fruits featured in *Handa's Surprise*
- Cutting board and knife
- Serving bowl and utensils
- Small plates
- Clean hands
- Plastic gloves

◆ I Will Never Not Ever Eat a Tomato

Child, L. (2003). *I will never not ever eat a tomato*. Cambridge, Mass: Candlewick Press.

Lola is a fussy eater until her big brother Charlie makes up inventive names for vegetables and other foods. Carrots become "orange twiglets from Jupiter," peas are "green drops from Greenland" and mashed potatoes turn into "cloud fluff from the pointiest peak of Mount Fuji."

ACTIVITY

▲ Ask children to list some of their favorite foods. Next, ask them to make up inventive names for the foods and use the words to write their own creative story.

♦ **In the Garden with Dr. Carver**

Grigsby, S. (2010). *In the garden with Doctor Carver.* Chicago, Ill: Albert Whitman. This historical fiction title for young readers features the famous plant scientist, George Washington Carver. It tells the story of how he took his "movable school," an old wagon pulled by a mule, to teach rural Alabamians how to grow food in their depleted soil. In this story, he visits a school and teaches Sally and the other children about nature and agriculture. This book is a great selection because it integrates food, history, culture and science into a beautifully illustrated and well-written story for children.

ACTIVITIES

▲ Two of the foods that Dr. George Washington Carver was known for were sweet potatoes and peanuts. He actually invented hundreds of uses (both food and non-food) for these products. Because sweet potatoes are a nutrient-rich vegetable, they make an ideal food for a tasting activity. Show students the sweet potatoes in their whole form and then prepare by scrubbing, poking with a knife and microwaving for 7-10 minutes on high or until tender (times vary with size of potatoes and power of the microwave). Allow to cool and cut into small pieces for tasting. Discuss different ways to prepare and enjoy sweet potatoes, including in mixed dishes, mashed, and seasoned with cinnamon, curry or other spices. Ask students whether their families eat sweet potatoes and how they are usually prepared in their homes.

You Will Need:

♦ Sweet Potatoes (1 large potato per 6-8 students)

♦ Vegetable Brush

♦ Sharp knife

♦ Microwave oven

♦ Small plates and forks

♦ Clean hands

♦ Plastic gloves

Discuss the importance of healthy soil for healthy plants. This is a great tie-in with school gardening projects such as composting, crop rotation and the importance of adding organic matter to soil to keep it healthy. If you do not have a school garden, start a growing project indoors. Herbs such as basil, chives, cilantro and dill are easy plants to grow in a sunny window.

◆ **Junie B., First Grader: Boss of Lunch** 🔟

Park, B. (2003). *Junie B., first grader: boss of lunch.* New York: Scholastic. In this Junie B. adventure, she is making trouble in the cafeteria. This hilarious book is supportive of the school meal program and sheds a positive light on "cafeteria ladies."

ACTIVITY

▲ Invite the cafeteria manager or food service director to the classroom to discuss how the school breakfast and lunch menus are designed to meet the nutritional needs of students. End the lesson by taking a field trip to the school kitchen.

◆ **Oliver's Milkshake**

French, V. & Bartlett, A. (2000). *Oliver's Milkshake.* London: Hodder Children's Books. In this story, picky eater Oliver visits a dairy farm with his aunt and cousin. They make a delicious milkshake from fresh milk, blueberries, a banana and ice.

ACTIVITY

▲ Try the following fruit smoothie recipe:

So-Berry-Good Smoothies

Ingredients:

1 cup frozen berries (strawberries, blueberries or raspberries), rinsed

1 frozen banana, broken into chunks

1 cup nonfat Greek vanilla yogurt

1 cup fat-free or 1% milk

Combine all ingredients in the blender; process until smooth. Serve immediately. Makes 4 servings.

You Will Need:

♦ Ingredients for smoothie recipe (see text)

♦ Blender

♦ Small cups or glasses for tasting

Other "Oliver" Books to Check Out From the Library*

♦ French, V. (1996). *Oliver's vegetables.* S. l: Orchard.
Oliver doesn't like vegetables until he visits his Grandpa's farm and discovers a variety of fresh garden vegetables.

♦ French, V. (1998). *Oliver's fruit salad.* London: Hodder Children's.
Oliver likes the fruit grown on his Grandpa's farm but not the fruit from the market. He changes his mind when Grandpa comes to visit and they make a fruit salad.

*These books are out of print in the U.S.

♦ Rah,Rah Radishes!
Sayre, A. (2011). *Rah, rah, radishes! a vegetable chant*. New York: Beach Lane Books. Written in rhyme with vivid colored vegetable photos taken at a local farmer's market, this book brings great fun to learning about vegetables.

ACTIVITY

▲ This book makes a great prelude to a class field trip to a local farmer's market. Challenge students to find vegetables and fruits not featured in this book and write their own chants about the produce they select.

♦ Stone Soup
Brown, M. (1986). *Stone Soup*. New York: Aladdin Books. This is the classic story of how three hungry soldiers convince the peasants of a small village that soup made of stones is indeed hearty and delicious. As the soldiers begin heating up their soup of water and three polished stones, the peasants eagerly contribute ingredients, including a few carrots, some cabbage, a little barley, beef, potatoes and milk, until finally the soldiers declare the soup "fit for a King."

You Will Need:
♦ Slow cooker
♦ Clean stone
♦ Tomato or vegetable juice
♦ Water
♦ pepper, herbs, spices
♦ Assorted vegetables (from children)
♦ Soup ladle
♦ Bowls and spoons
♦ Clean hands
♦ Plastic gloves

ACTIVITY

▲ As a class, create a pot of vegetable stone soup, using a slow cooker and clean stone. Use tomato or vegetable juice and water for the base, add pepper, desired herbs and spices, and ask each child to bring a fresh vegetable from home. Assemble first thing in the morning, cook on high and eat for a snack during the later part of the school day.

♦ The Berenstain Bears and Too Much Junk Food
Berenstain, S. & Berenstain, J. (1985). *The Berenstain Bears and Too Much Junk Food*. New York: Random House.
When Mama Bear notices her two cubs getting a little chubby, she decides to curtail their junk food habits. To his surprise and dismay, Papa

Bear must forgo much of his junk food and sugary beverages as well. Great family reading, the Berenstains do an excellent job of covering basic nutrition principles, the importance of a healthy lifestyle and the role exercise plays in good health.

ACTIVITIES

▲ Ask each child to write down or draw pictures of physical activities that his or her family can do together.

▲ Lead a discussion on how exercise and nutrition work together to produce fit young bodies. See chapter 11 for more ideas.

◆ The Hatseller and the Monkeys

Diakité, B. (1999). *The Hatseller and the Monkeys*. New York: Scholastic Press. In this West African version of a popular folktale, hatseller Ba-Musa forgets to eat breakfast before he takes off on a day-long journey. He soon falls asleep under a mango tree and the monkeys make off with his hats. Only after he eats is he able to think clearly and devise a way to get his hats back.

ACTIVITIES

▲ Ask students to write a story or draw a picture about the importance of breakfast and how it "wakes up the brain," helping them to think, focus and learn at school.

▨ Have students create a "Good Morning" breakfast place mat out of construction paper, magazine pictures or their own art that illustrates the importance of a healthy breakfast.

▲ Hold a mango tasting. Demonstrate how to peel and slice a fresh mango, show children the long oblong seed and pass out samples to taste.

You Will Need:
◆ Mangos
◆ Sharp knife
◆ Small plates for tasting
◆ Clean hands
◆ Plastic gloves

◆ The Little Red Hen

Ottolenghi, C. (2002). *The little red hen.* Columbus, Ohio: McGraw-Hill Children's Pub. While this classic tale sends a strong message about work, cooperation and consequences, an underlying theme teaches children the stages of bread production. From wheat seed to bread, the Little Red Hen perseveres in her production of a loaf of bread.

ACTIVITIES

▲ Use visual props and a baking activity to tell the story. Obtain wheat kernels (purchase from mills or the bulk section of grocery stores), stalks of dried wheat (available in craft stores), whole wheat flour and whole wheat bread or roll dough (made from scratch or purchased frozen). Show students the props as you read the story. After the story, divide the bread dough into roll-sized portions for each student. Encourage children to create their own "bread art" by kneading and shaping the dough. Line a baking tray with parchment baking paper, label each child's bread art, bake according to package or recipe instructions and serve as a snack. (It's a good idea to enlist the help of your cafeteria manager with this project.)

You Will Need:
◆ Wheat kernels
◆ Dried wheat stalks
◆ Whole wheat flour
◆ Whole wheat bread dough
◆ Clean work surface
◆ Parchment baking paper
◆ Baking trays
◆ Oven
◆ Napkins or small plates
◆ Clean hands
◆ Plastic gloves

Using potting soil and small containers, have students plant the wheat kernels and care for their plants. If you have a school garden, you can also designate a raised bed or area to grow wheat. See Chapter 7 for more on growing plants.

◆ **The Little Red Hen (Makes a Pizza!)**

Sturges, P. (2002). *The little red hen (makes a pizza).* New York: Puffin Books. The industrious Little Red Hen is back with a modern spin! This whimsical and updated version is entertaining and also a good excuse to make a healthy pizza from scratch.

ACTIVITY

▲As a class, make "perfectly personal pizzas," the recipe activity featured on page 96.

◆ **The Very Hungry Caterpillar**

Carle, E. (1994). The *Very Hungry Caterpillar*. New York: Philomel Books. This story clearly and vividly illustrates how food is needed to build young bodies. The caterpillar, with his insatiable appetite, eventually grows big and prepares to turn into a beautiful butterfly. This book sets the stage for a discussion of how food fuels the growth of all living things, even kids.

ACTIVITIES

▲ Encourage children to create a story about "The Very Hungry Kid," complete with the foods they (or the character they create) would choose to eat on each day of the week and the resultant growth that occurs.

▲ To measure how food fuels the growth of children, start a classroom growth chart. Take height measurements each month, noting the changes as the year progresses. Be sure to point out that all children grow differently and there is no one single "best" size, shape or growth pattern because we are individuals.

◆ **Two Old Potatoes and Me**

Coy, J. & Fisher, C. (2009). *Two Old Potatoes and Me*. New York: Dragonfly Books. A father and daughter find two old potatoes in a cupboard and learn how this vegetable grows by planting the potato "eyes" in their backyard. They weed, water, wait and follow the growing season to see if they will get new potatoes.

ACTIVITIES

▲ Potatoes provide a powerhouse of nutrients, including potassium, fiber, vitamin C and more. As long as potatoes are not deep fried or smothered in butter or other fats, they are a very nutritious vegetable. Ask students to brainstorm healthy ways to eat potatoes. (HINT: Serve baked, broiled, roasted or steamed; Use small amounts of cheese, guacamole, fat-free Greek yogurt with chives, or salsa as toppings.)

🌱 Have students plant potato eyes in containers or the school garden and monitor and record their results.

UPPER ELEMENTARY (THIRD-FIFTH GRADES)

♦ Janey Junkfood's Fresh Adventure!

Storper, B. (2011). *Janey Junkfood's fresh adventure! Making Good Eating Great Fun!* Hatfield, MA: FoodPlay Productions.

Written by Barbara Storper, the dietitian who created the award-winning theater company FoodPlay, this book uses a colorful scrapbook-style format to teach children how to decipher food labels, the importance of eating breakfast, the effects of a junk food diet, fun ways to enjoy fruits and vegetables and more. Children follow Ace Food Detective Tobe Fit as she discovers that healthy eating habits are the missing ingredient to Janey's success at making the National Junior Juggling Team.

ACTIVITIES

▲ Visit the FoodPlay website at http://www.foodplay.com to download a companion activity guide with discussion questions, teaching ideas, and activity sheets.

♦ Nothing's Fair in Fifth Grade

DeClements, B. (2009). *Nothing's fair in fifth grade.* New York, N.Y: Puffin Books (reissued edition). Written by a school counselor, this fictional story explores the psychological issues surrounding childhood obesity. Not only is Elsie Edwards the new girl at school, she is also obese and considered "gross" by classmates. This book teaches valuable lessons about the prejudice, bullying and outright cruelty endured by overweight people in our society. **Note:** This book was originally written in the 1980s so historical references are out-of-date.

ACTIVITY

▲ Lead a discussion on how people come in a variety of shapes and sizes, pointing out that there is no one "best" way to look. This is also a good opportunity to discuss bullying in all its forms and strategies for dealing with this hurtful and inappropriate behavior. You may want to invite the school counselor to join your classroom in this discussion.

◆ Pig and the Shrink

Todd, P. (2000). *Pig and the shrink.* New York: Dell Yearling. *(note: this book is out of print, check in libraries or from online sellers)*
Tucker learns about life, friendship and ambition when he decides to use "Pig" (Angelo Pighetti) as his science project. Pig is overweight and frequently picked on by classmates. Tucker's efforts at changing Pig's eating habits backfire, Pig gains even more weight during the experiment and Tucker fears he has lost a good friend. This humorous book sends a strong message about acceptance.

ACTIVITY

▲ Discuss with students the ethics of changing people because you want them to change. Use some or all of the following questions for discussion:
  – Is it acceptable to tell another person what to eat?
  – Do you want someone else to control your eating or exercise habits?
  – Is there a way to help people without forcing them to change?
Ask students to note the difference between helping a friend and hurting a friend. Suggest they write in a journal about how they would help friends with nutrition or weight problems.

◆ What's Cooking, Jenny Archer?

Conford, E. (2006). *What's Cooking, Jenny Archer?* Little, Brown Young Readers. A "creative" cook who enjoys sandwiches made with mint jelly and bologna on raisin bread, Jenny begins concocting her own lunches for school. Soon her friends want her to make their lunches, too. Figuring she will quickly get rich, Jenny sets out to sell creative lunches to her friends. Her plan backfires when she is unable to please the picky palates of her friends.

ACTIVITIES

▲ Create an original "*MyPlate* sandwich." (See page 59.)

🍽 Invite the cafeteria manager or food service director to discuss how he or she manages to meet the tastes and preferences of all the children in the school. Suggest that the class assist the manager in planning a school breakfast or lunch menu.

Nonfiction Food & Nutrition Books for Upper Elementary

♦ Charney, S., Goldbeck, D. & Larson, M. (2007). *The ABCs of fruits and vegetables and beyond.* Woodstock: Ceres Press.
This is really two books in one. The first half of the book is geared towards early childhood and includes colorful visuals with clever rhymes. The second half – the "beyond" section – is packed with information, trivia, geography, recipes and website/book recommendations that will be of interest to the upper elementary student.

♦ Pollan, M. (2009). *The omnivore's dilemma for kids: the secrets behind what you eat.* New York: Dial Books.
This book is a great classroom reference for advanced students who want to delve more deeply into the complex issues surrounding food and agriculture. While billed as a book for ages 10 and up, it is geared more towards the adolescent reader.

♦ Shanley, E. & Thompson, C. (2011). *Fueling the teen machine : what it takes to make good choices for yourself every day.* Boulder, Colo: Bull Pub. Co.
Although focused on adolescents, this is an appropriate nutrition reference book for upper elementary and middle school students. It has not yet been updated with the *MyPlate* food guide.

Putting a Nutrition Twist on Fairy Tales

Once upon a time, there was an enchanted school cafeteria where the princess ate her peas, the porridge was always "just right," a vegetarian wolf never bothered the three little pigs and the breakfast eggs were laid by a prized golden goose.

A fun activity that sharpens writing, illustrating, storytelling and comprehension skills is to retell classic stories, adding a nutritional bent. The possibilities for student assignments are endless. Below are a few examples.

ACTIVITIES

▲ Remember Jack Sprat, the one who ate no fat while his wife would eat no lean? What would you tell Jack and Mrs. Sprat about nutritional moderation?

▲ Write a letter to "Baby Bear," giving him ideas on added ingredients that would make his porridge extra delicious and nutritious.

▲ If Little Red Riding Hood were really concerned about her sick grandmother's health, what "goodies" should she pack in the basket that would help Granny recover and stay healthy?

▲ Imagine that the witch in "Hansel and Gretel" was actually a good and caring witch, concerned with the nutritional health of the children who came to visit. Instead of gingerbread and candy, of what foods would her house be made?

▲ In the story of the grasshopper and the ant, the ant stocked up for the winter while the grasshopper failed to plan and went hungry. What advice would you give the grasshopper on collecting and storing food for the winter?

Children's tales with a reference to food or eating

Traditional Stories
Goldilocks and the Three Bears
Jack and the Beanstalk
Little Red Riding Hood
The Little Gingerbread Man

Aesop's Fables
The Ant and the Grasshopper
The Fox and the Grapes
The Town Mouse and the
 Country Mouse
The Goose with the Golden Eggs

Grimm's Fairy Tales
Cinderella
Hansel and Gretel
Snow White

Mother Goose's Nursery Rhymes
The Old Woman Who Lived
 in a Shoe
Hey diddle, diddle
Old Mother Hubbard
Sing a Song of Sixpence
Peter Piper
Jack Sprat
Little Miss Muffet
This Little Pig Went to Market

American Tales
Johnny Appleseed
Paul Bunyan

▲ The story of "Jack and the Beanstalk" fails to tell about the crop of beans that must have resulted from such a large plant. Write or tell about what Jack and his mom did with all those beans. Were they green beans or dried beans? Did they eat them or sell them? How did they cook them? Any recipe ideas?

▲ When Winnie-the-Pooh indulges himself with too much honey and condensed milk at Rabbit's house, he gets stuck attempting to exit

Rabbit's hole. How could Pooh Bear improve his eating and exercise habits so he doesn't get stuck the next time?

⊕ Ask students to develop storybook names for cafeteria menu items served during the month. Examples include Peter Piper's Pepper Pizza, Jack Sprat's low-Fat Ranch Dressing, Three Bear Breakfast Porridge Bar (with hot and cold cereals), Little Miss Muffet's Muffins (good served with curds and whey, or milk and yogurt if you insist), Jack Horner's Fresh Plums (sans thumb, thank you) or Jack-and-the-Beanstalk's Best Baked Beans.

Descriptive Writing

Using food as a subject is an effective way to develop descriptive writing skills. While children may have limited experience in other areas, they encounter food several times each day. The novice writer can more easily describe scenes and objects that are based on firsthand experience. A few ideas are described below.

ACTIVITIES

▲ The sight, smell and taste of food can evoke strong emotions. Suggest that students write about a particular meal or food that made them feel especially happy, excited, sentimental, sad, grouchy or even angry. Encourage them to provide details regarding the surroundings, people, food and why they felt as they did.

▲ Bring in colorful pictures, posters or samples of real food. Assign students the task of describing one food, using as many details as possible.

▲ Bring in various foods for a snack or tasting. Ask students to write down how different foods appeal to each of their five senses. A few examples: "The strawberry is a beautiful, red color with seeds that remind me of polka dots." "When I bite into a carrot, the crunchy sound fills up my whole head." "The smell of fresh bread makes me feel warm and happy clear down to my toes."

> **You Will Need:**
> ◆ Colorful food pictures
>
> OR
>
> ◆ A variety of real food samples to observe, smell and taste

Writing Activities for the Young Nutrition Advocate

Starting at a young age, it is important for kids to learn to voice their opinions about the policies and messages that affect their nutrition choices. The goal of writing letters should be to communicate opinions in a clear, constructive manner. Two areas to target include school meals and food advertisements. You can also encourage your students to contact their legislators about laws that influence food and nutrition issues and policies. For contact information, see http://www.usa.gov/Contact/Elected.shtml.

SCHOOL MEALS

ACTIVITIES

▲ Begin by writing letters to the cafeteria manager or district food service director. Suggest that children begin the letter by stating what they like best about the school meals. If there are comments, suggestions or criticisms, word them in a constructive way (e.g., "One change I would like to see in the menu/cafeteria is _____" or "My idea of the perfect school breakfast/lunch menu is _____.").

▲ Write or send an email to the United States Department of Agriculture (USDA), the federal agency that oversees child nutrition programs, including school breakfast, lunch and summer feeding programs. Communicate what you like the best about the school meal program and changes that you would like to see implemented. Address your letters to:

USDA Food and Nutrition Service

3101 Park Center Drive

Alexandria, Virginia 22302

If you would like to send an email regarding the child nutrition programs, you can visit the USDA food and nutrition service website at http://www.fns.usda.gov/cnd. Click on "contact us" and it will give you a list to choose from. You can send an email to the national offices or to your state child nutrition office.

FOOD ADVERTISEMENTS

ACTIVITIES

▲ The next time you are watching television on Saturday morning, keep a list of the advertised foods that fall into the "empty calorie" category such as candy, sweetened beverages, sugary cereal or fatty fast food meals. Also keep a list of ads for healthful foods from the five food groups. Are there more ads for healthful foods or low-nutrition foods? (See worksheet on page 143.) You can write letters to those responsible for the ads, including the food company who pays for the advertising or the television network that accepts the advertising.

Don't Buy It!
An engaging website for kids is the *Don't Buy it: Get Media Smart* site from PBS Kids located at:
http://pbskids.org/dontbuyit

To find the address for the food company, look at the food container in question the next time you go to the grocery store (or ask an adult to do it for you). Printed on the can, bottle or package is a mailing address and often, a website address. If you visit the website, look for a link that says "contact us" and use the contact form to write and submit your opinion.

▲ Write or send an email to the television networks and let them know how you feel about their food advertising. The major networks can be reached at the addresses listed below. To send an email, go to the network website and find the "contact us" link.

ABC
Audience Relations Dept.
500 S. Buena Vista St.
Burbank, CA 91521-4551
Web: www.abc.com

NBC
Viewer Services
30 Rockefeller Plaza
New York, NY 10112
Web: www.nbc.com

CBS
Audience Services
51 W. 52nd Street
New York, NY 10019
Web: www.cbs.com

Fox Broadcasting Company
Fox Viewer Services
P.O. Box 900
Beverly Hills, CA 90213
Web: www.foxworld.com

PBS
PBS Viewer Mail
1320 Braddock Place
Alexandria, VA 22314-1698
Web: www.pbs.org

Nickelodeon
Viewer Services
1515 Broadway
New York, NY 10036
Web: www.nick.com

Discovery Channel
Viewer Relations
7700 Wisconsin Avenue
Bethesda, MD 20814
Web: www.discovery.com

Disney Channel
3800 West Almada Avenue
Burbank, CA 91505
Web:
http://disneychannel.disney.go.com

You can also file a complaint by contacting the Children's Advertising Review Unit, a division of the Better Business Bureau:

Children's Advertising Review Unit
70 West 36th Street, 12th Floor
New York, NY 10018
Web: http://www.caru.org

Spelling List

Include food, nutrition and fitness words in your list of weekly spelling words. Examples are listed below.

Aerobic	Fiber	Mineral
Calorie	Fitness	Nutrient
Carbohydrate	Flexibility	Nutrition
Dairy	Fruit	Protein
Diet	Grain	Strength
Dietitian	Growth	Vegetable
Energy	Healthy	Vitamin
Exercise	Hydration	Water

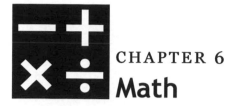

CHAPTER 6

Math

"I liked it when you showed us how much fat and sugar were in those two lunches. I was surprised when you showed us how much fat was in the lunch with the Big Mac. I thought that was kind of gross." —Dawn

Whether counting daily servings from the *MyPlate* food groups, calculating nutrients in a recipe or learning how to decipher the *Nutrition Facts* food label, the application of nutrition requires basic math skills. Likewise, math skills can be learned and reinforced through the use of real-life food activities such as following and devising recipes, dividing up portions or making purchases at the grocery store.

One food related math skill that comes naturally to children, even the very young, is division. Children think of it as "fair share" and are always mindful that they get their deserved allotment of animal crackers, grapes or cheese chunks. Build this natural inclination into a snacktime math lesson. For example, ask students to first count the number of fresh-cut pineapple chunks in a bowl (use two bowls and transfer as they count). Say, for example, a group of five children counted 30 chunks of pineapple. In the next step, ask the students this question: "There are 30 chunks of pineapple in this bowl and there are five of you, so how many do you each get?" Conversely, ask children how many whole grain crackers you need to buy if each student typically eats four squares. The children have unknowingly applied both basic division and multiplication while snacking on healthy foods.

Teaching Label Lessons

Reading and understanding food labels helps children sharpen their nutrition, math and critical thinking skills. The following activities will help children interpret and apply the *Nutrition Facts* label information.

Spot the Block

The U.S. Food and Drug Administration (FDA) has a "Spot the Block" campaign to increase *Nutrition Facts* label literacy. Aimed at 9-13 year-olds, the site challenges tweens and their parents to use the *Nutrition Facts* Label (the "block") to make healthy food choices. http://1.usa.gov/xlXXBO

Table 6-1

Highlights of the Nutrition Facts Food Label

The *Nutrition Facts* food label makes it easy for kids to decipher the sugar content of fruit drinks, compare the sodium in different varieties of deli meat or check the fiber in breakfast cereal. A *Nutrition Facts* label is required on most packaged foods. The following points will help you to decipher label information and enable you to be a better "food fact finder."

▲ The first thing to look at on a label is the serving size and number of servings per container. What appears to be a "single serving" container can often contain two to three servings.

▲ Labels generally highlight four key nutrients including vitamins A and C, calcium and iron. If a food is naturally high in one or more of these key nutrients, it is likely a source of several other nutrients as well. Manufacturers may include information on additional nutrients on a voluntary basis.

▲ Labels include values for total carbohydrate, as well as a breakdown of the carbohydrates derived from sugar and dietary fiber. It's important to note that the sugar value includes naturally occurring sugars (e.g. fruit and milk) as well as added sugars.

▲ The *Nutrition Facts* label makes it easy to calculate the percentage of calories from fat in a food product. (See Table 6-2 for calculation). Keep in mind, though, that the goal to slide under 35 percent calories from fat applies to the diet over the course of the day and not to individual foods.

▲ The % Daily Value (%DV) helps you figure out whether a food is low or high in a nutrient. The 5-10-20 rule is helpful when looking at a serving of food:
♦ 5% or less is considered a low amount.
♦ 10% means the food is a "good source" of that nutrient.
♦ 20% means that the food is high in that nutrient.
Be careful though, because sometimes highly processed foods have been fortified with nutrients in order to make them appear more nutritious.

▲ *Nutrition Facts* labels include a chart with the daily recommended levels for fats, cholesterol, sodium, carbohydrate and fiber at reference values of 2,000 and 2,500 calories. Depending on age, gender and activity level, children typically require between 1400 – 2200 calories each day. The personalized *Daily Food Plan* at choosemyplate.gov identifies a specific calorie estimate.

▲ Food labels are required to contain complete ingredient lists The ingredients are listed from most to least, by weight. This feature is especially important for those who have allergies or sensitivities to specific food additives.

▲ For more information and updates on *Nutrition Facts* food labels, visit the FDA food labeling and nutrition website at http://1.usa.gov/xQZe34

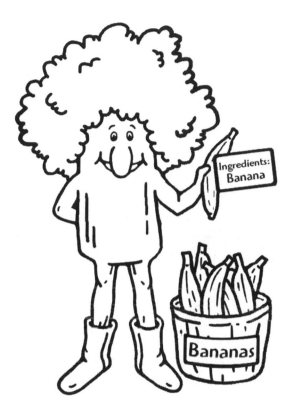

Because produce and seafood aren't packaged, they don't come with a product label. The FDA has a voluntary *Nutrition Facts* program for fresh fruit, fresh vegetables and fresh seafood. You may have seen the posters in the grocery store which feature the 20 most frequently consumed raw fruits, vegetables and seafood in the United States. The posters can also be downloaded from the FDA website at http://1.usa.gov/yojFax.

ACTIVITIES

▲ DESIGN A "FRONT PACK" NUTRITION LABEL

Many food companies have added nutrition labeling symbols or other information on the front of food packages. There has been a lot of debate and controversy about which information food companies should put on these "front pack" labels. Some experts worry that companies are trying to mislead and confuse consumers with this additional labeling.

Break students into small groups and have them brainstorm and design a front-pack food product label, emphasizing both the content as well as the design. Ask students whether they think it is better to focus on the positive nutrients such as fiber, vitamins, minerals and protein or if the label should serve as a warning for high levels of sugar, fat, or sodium. Encourage creativity in the design of the food package, challenging students to come up with a label that is both eye-catching and easy to understand.

▲ WHAT'S YOUR SERVING SIZE?

The serving size listed on a product label is often different from what we think of as a "helping." To make this point, bring in a large box of breakfast cereal, cereal bowls and measuring cups. Cover or remove the *Nutrition Facts* label information from the box. Ask children, a few at a time, to pour themselves a "bowl of ce-

You Will Need:
- Box of cereal
- Cereal bowl
- Measuring cups

real," typical of what they would eat for breakfast or a snack. Next, have students measure and record how much they poured into the bowl. After everyone has taken a turn, appoint one child to read aloud the serving amount listed on the label. Ask how many children measured the same amount, more or less than the label serving size. Remind students that the nutrition information on the label pertains to the standard label serving size. Ask what that means in different situations (e.g. "If a label lists 4 grams of dietary fiber and your serving size is half as much as the standard serving, how many grams of fiber did you eat?" or "If a label indicates there are 12 grams of sugar in one serving but you ate 1 ½ servings, how much sugar did you actually eat?")

Nutrition Facts

Serving Size 1 cup (228g)
Servings Per Container about 2

Amount Per Serving

Calories 250   Calories from Fat 110

% Daily Value*

Total Fat 12g	**18%**
Saturated Fat 3g	**15%**
Trans Fat 0g	
Cholesterol 30mg	**10%**
Sodium 470mg	**20%**
Total Carbohydrate 31g	**10%**
Dietary Fiber 0g	**0%**
Sugars 5g	
Proteins 5g	

Vitamin A	4%
Vitamin C	2%
Calcium	20%
Iron	4%

* Percent Daily Values are based on a 2,000 calorie diet. Your Daily Values may be higher or lower depending on your calorie needs:

	Calories:	2,000	2,500
Total Fat	Less than	65g	80g
Saturated Fat	Less than	20g	25g
Cholesterol	Less than	300mg	300mg
Sodium	Less than	2,400mg	2,400mg
Total Carbohydrate		300g	375g
Dietary Fiber		25g	30g

Source: U.S. Food and Drug Administration

Going Further: Make a class graph that visually shows individual differences in serving sizes. Have each student plot his or her serving amount on a poster-sized bar graph. Include a comparison bar that shows the serving size listed on the label.

▲ CALORIES FROM SUGAR AND FAT

Calories in food come from carbohydrate (in the form of starches or sugar), protein or fat. When gauging the nutritional merit of a food item, it is often helpful to look at the total grams of sugar as well as the number of calories that come from fat. While whole, unprocessed foods such as fruit and milk contain natural sugars, most of the sugar in our food supply comes from added sugars. The American Heart Association advises a daily limit of 6-9 teaspoons (24-36 grams) of added sugar. Most Americans eat far more than this limit.

In regards to fats, it is important to note that all fat sources contain the same amount of calories (9 per gram) but some fats are better choices for health. Canola oil, olive oil, avocados, olives and nuts are examples of more healthful fat sources while saturated fats and trans fats should be limited. See page 171 for more about fat.

What about trans fats?

♦ Trans fatty acids are formed when food manufacturers hydrogenate vegetable oil to make it more solid. Trans fats are found in foods containing "partially hydrogenated" vegetable oils. Examples include certain margarines, baked goods, snack foods and many other processed foods.

♦ Trans fats have been shown to raise blood cholesterol levels and contribute to the development of heart disease. Most nutrition experts recommend limiting the intake of trans fat as much as possible. Food manufacturers are required to list the amount of trans fat on every food that carries a *Nutrition Facts* label.

♦ Labeling laws allow a product with less than .5 gram trans fat/serving to declare it as zero on the label. This is misleading because a product may still contain some trans fat. It is important to read the ingredient list and limit or avoid foods that contain partially hydrogenated oils.

"Calories from Fat" is listed next to "Calories" on the *Nutrition Facts* label. Over the course of a day, the recommended goal for children ages 4-18 is to eat a range of 25 to 35 percent of calories from fat. Not every food needs to fall below the 35 percent maximum. Foods higher in fat can be balanced with lower fat foods to obtain a daily average that is under 35 percent. Using the *Nutrition Facts* label, encourage students to calculate the percentage of calories from fat in several food products (refer to Table 6-2).

Note: Since students don't always have access to calculators, pencils or paper, encourage the use of estimation in evaluating the nutrition content of foods. For example, the estimated fat content of a package of cookies with 65 calories per serving and 35 calories from fat would be "slightly more than one-half of the calories."

Table 6-2

Calculating Percent Calories from Fat

To calculate percent calories from fat using the *Nutrition Facts* food label, you need the **Calories** and **Calories from Fat** from the label. Simply divide calories from fat by the calories and multiply by 100 to arrive at the percentage.

The equation looks like this:
(Calories From Fat ÷ Calories) x 100 = % Calories From Fat

Example: A box of snack crackers provides 80 **calories** for a serving of 5 crackers. The **calories from fat** are listed as 20.
(20 ÷ 80) x 100 = 25% Calories From Fat

▲ MAKING COMPARISONS

The food label is a powerful tool for comparing similar food products. Younger children can begin by comparing one nutrient in different products, while students in the intermediate grades can learn to compare several parameters on a label. Suggest that students develop graphs or pictures with fractional pieces to illustrate the differences between foods.

Ten suggestions for comparing labels, ranked from simple to more complex, are listed below.

1. Sugar in Breakfast Cereal: Bring in a variety of cereal boxes. Locate "Sugars" on the label. On a piece of paper, rank the cereals in order of sugar content.

2. Total Fat in Crackers: Rank various crackers in order of "total fat" content.

You Will Need:
♦ A variety of food labels

OR

♦ Observation and recording of label information during a field trip to a grocery store

3. Sodium in Snack Foods: Compare the sodium content in one serving of pretzels, chips, packaged popcorn and snack crackers.

4. Fiber in Bread: Just because bread is dark in color, it's not necessarily whole grain or full of fiber (it may have molasses or caramel coloring added to make it darker). Because the refining process removes most of the naturally occurring nutrients, "enriched flour" is simply refined white flour with a few added nutrients. Compare the dietary fiber content per serving of white bread, 100 percent whole wheat bread and bread made primarily with enriched flour that is simply labeled "wheat."

5. Sugars in Unlikely Places: Various forms of sugar are commonly added to processed foods, even those we don't think of as sweet. Send children on a scavenger hunt for foods that contain added sugars, such as ketchup, spaghetti sauce, mayonnaise, baked beans, hot dogs and certain breads.

> **Be a Sugar Sleuth**
> There are many ways to say "sugar" on food labels. All of the following are forms of sugar:
> - High fructose corn syrup
> - Sucrose
> - Dextrose
> - Glucose
> - Molasses
> - Honey
> - Brown sugar
> - Corn sweetener
> - Corn syrup
> - Fructose
> - Invert sugar
> - Fruit juice concentrates

6. Rating Lunch Meats: There is a notable difference in the fat, calorie and sodium content of luncheon meats. For homework or as part of a class field trip, assign students the task of finding and comparing at least five different lunch meats (e.g., lean ham or roast beef, different types of turkey meat, bologna and salami). Note the difference in calories, fat and sodium for a standard serving size. Which products are the best overall choices?

7. The Merits of Milk: "Two percent" milk sounds like it must be low in fat, but is it? Write down the total fat, calories and calories from fat for fat-free, 1%, 2% and whole milk. Have students calculate the percent calories from fat in all four milks. Ask students why milk listed as 1% or 2% fat appears much higher in fat when using the percent calories from fat calculation. (ANSWER: 1% or 2% refers to fat by weight, which is low since most of the weight in milk comes from water.)

> **Going Further:**
>
> Compare the calcium content among different varieties of milk or compare the fat, sugar and calorie content of various frozen desserts such as ice cream, frozen yogurt, sherbet and sorbet.

8. Finding the "Better Butter": Although spreads such as butter, butter blends and margarines are, by nature, mostly fat, the key nutritional difference is the amount of fat that derives from either trans fat or saturated fat. Both trans fats and saturated fats are associated with higher blood cholesterol and an increased risk for heart disease in later life. See pg. 88 for more about trans fats.

Ask children to look at a variety of labels and rank them by the level of trans and saturated fats. Note that there is a large difference in the saturated fat content of liquid, soft tub and stick margarines and spreads. Students will discover that certain margarines and spreads have nearly as much saturated fat as butter.

Keep in mind, too, that the flavor of butter is preferred by many, especially chefs and those involved in fine food preparation. Their advice: Use real butter — just use less of it!

9. Noodle Know-How: Kids may be surprised to learn that many brands of ramen noodles fare worse in fat and sodium content than an average serving of potato chips. Encourage students to read and evaluate their favorite ramen noodle labels. Ask them to look for brands that are lower in fat during their next trip to the grocery store.

> **Going Further:** Ask students how the nutrition of ramen noodles compares to standard egg noodles.

10. Taking a Closer Look at So-Called Fruit Snacks: If you believe the advertising and packaging, there are a whole array of processed "fruit snacks" just loaded with fruit. To dispel this myth, teach students how to read ingredient labels on packaged foods, pointing out that ingredients are listed from most to least, by weight. Ask them to read the ingredient labels on a variety of fruit snacks to see in what order actual fruit falls in the ingredient list (if it appears at all!). Often, fruit is listed as the third or fourth ingredient, behind various types of sugar, corn syrup and gelatin.

Measuring Nutrients in Food

Children can best grasp the concept of "high fat" or "high sugar" when they can actually see the fat and sugar in a food. The activities below give students practice in weighing and measuring, provide reference for what a gram is and visually display the fat and sugar content of various foods.

ACTIVITIES

▲ WHAT'S A GRAM?

Nutrient information on food labels, recipes, restaurant brochures and reference tables is mostly metric, with food components measured in grams and milligrams (1/1000 of a gram). Some nutrients, such as vitamin K and iodine, are needed in such small amounts that they are measured in micrograms (that's one millionth of a gram!).

> **You Will Need:**
> - Gram scale
> - Paper clip and other small items
> - Soda pop label
> - Coffee filters
> - Sugar

The weight of a gram is approximately that of a small paper clip. Using a gram scale, ask students to weigh different common items such as a paper clip, pencil, eraser or chalk.

Next, explain how the weights of many of the nutrients in foods are also listed in grams. The average 12-ounce can of soda pop, for instance, contains about 40 grams of sugar. To demonstrate, first place a coffee filter on top of the scale. Next, show the students how to "zero" the scale. Fill the coffee filter with sugar until the scale registers 40 grams, resulting in a small mountain of sugar!

▲ SETTING UP A CENTER

To set up a center for students to weigh and measure the fat and sugar in foods, you will need a gram scale, teaspoons, one pound of sugar, one pound of vegetable shortening, coffee filters, small plastic plates and food packages or labels.

Another way to measure grams is to use a teaspoon. A teaspoon of sugar or fat weighs approximately 4 grams, so students can measure the teaspoons of fat and sugar in food by dividing the total grams by 4.

On a long table, set out a variety of food packages or labels. Examples include candy bars, cereal bars, yogurt containers, cereal boxes, potato chips, pretzels, crackers, cookies, beverage containers and fast food containers (nutrient information, including fat and sugar content, is usually available in the restaurant or at the restaurant's website).

A few at a time, students will read the labels and measure the fat and sugar content of the different food items, using coffee filters for sugar and plastic plates for fat. Have them place the containers with fat and sugar in front of each food package or label until they have measured all foods. When they are done, instruct them to scoop the fat and sugar back into the original containers and allow another group of students to work the center. (NOTE: Plastic plates can be washed and reused many times.)

Going Further:

- Consider a semi-permanent display of the fat and sugar in foods for the classroom or cafeteria. Invite other classes to observe and comment.

- Using food labels, measure the fiber content (in grams) in a variety of breads and cereals, using bran cereal to represent the fiber.

Graphing

A visual way to present and evaluate information is through the use of graphing. Nutrition goals, trends and concepts become more meaningful when children can see them plotted on a graph. Graph paper, colored pencils or markers and a ruler are all that is needed to complete the following bar or line graphs.

ACTIVITIES

▲ Using a completed one-day food record, explain how to count servings and graph daily food intake. After counting the number of servings from each of the five food groups and "extras," students can compare foods eaten to the recommended servings in *MyPlate*. Ask students to explain what the graph shows about their diets. Based on the results, suggest they set personal nutrition goals.

▲ Have students graph personal nutrition or fitness goals. Examples include eating three cups of vegetables each day, limiting candy to one serving a day or bike riding at least twenty minutes daily. The vertical axis should include numbers from 0 to 10 (for number of servings) or 0 to 60 minutes (for minutes spent bicycling). Place a red dot or line at the level of the goal (if a bar graph, draw a red bar that represents the goal). Underneath it, label it "Goal." Along the horizontal axis, write the days of the week.

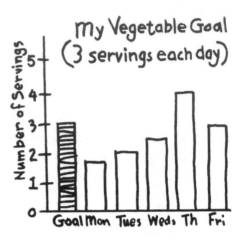

Each day, keep track of how many servings or minutes. Plot results on the graph above the appropriate date. For line graphs, connect the dots to make a line. Ask students to explain their graphs and report progress in meeting their goals.

▲ Choose one food group and survey the class to find out how many servings from that food group they ate yesterday. Assign groups of students to graph the data in various ways. For example, ask how many servings of fruit were consumed. On the board, write down the number of servings eaten by each student. Ask one group to compare the number of servings eaten by girls compared to boys. Another group can compare fruit intake of students who ate the school meal versus those who brought a lunch from home. Still another can compare fruit servings by table or group. Other ideas include comparing students by birthday month, eye or hair color or whether their last name begins with a letter in the first or last half of the alphabet. (This activity is also a great way to reinforce skills in averaging numbers.)

Ask students to draw conclusions about the factors that might influence fruit intake in the class.

Going Further: Involve the entire school in this activity, assessing food intake in other classes and grade levels. You may even want to challenge another class to a "good nutrition" duel, setting goals, graphing progress and rewarding completed goals with small prizes or incentives.

Create a Recipe

Devising a recipe gives children a chance to develop measuring and writing skills, exercise their creativity and eat the results of their labor. They can also share their own recipes with family and friends or start their own personal cookbook. Below are some simple ideas for recipe development that result in a high rate of tasty success.

Note: Before you conduct any of the food activities recommended in this chapter, review Appendix A, "Guidelines for Safe Classroom Cooking." Make sure you communicate with parents and inquire about any food allergies, intolerances or medical conditions that will influence the foods that you can offer.

For each recipe, provide a clean table with measuring cups and spoons, scale (optional), plastic knives and spoons, paper and pencils, plastic gloves, bowls filled with ingredients and individual plates or bowls for students to create their recipes.

Have students work in pairs, one as the cook and one as the recorder. After each recipe is complete, the children will switch roles.

When creating a recipe, it is important to start small, measuring a small amount at a time and then adding more as needed. Remind students that they can always add more but they are not allowed to subtract. (It is not sanitary to dump ingredients back into the serving bowl.) Demonstrate how to accurately measure ingredients, using the plastic knife to level off the measuring cup or spoon. After students determine the "right" amount of an ingredient, the recorder's

You Will Need:

- Clean work space
- Measuring cups and spoons
- Scale (optional)
- Plastic knives and spoons
- Paper and pencils
- Plastic gloves
- Bowls filled with ingredients (see text)
- Individual plates or bowls

job is to write it down. Later at their desks, students can complete their recipes by adding instructions and illustrations.

▲ **TRAIL MIX:** Provide ingredients such as raisins, dried berries, other dried fruit (chopped, if needed), peanuts, almonds, pumpkin seeds, sunflower seeds, wheat germ and quick-cooking oatmeal.

▲ **YOGURT PARFAIT:** Use clear plastic cups to make the parfaits. Instruct children to layer their parfait as they wish, using such ingredients as fat-free lemon or vanilla yogurt, crushed walnuts or wheat germ, berries, banana slices and melon balls.

▲ **VEGETABLE SALAD:** Big on nutrition and easy to assemble, creating a vegetable salad recipe is one way to entice kids to eat vegetables. Include familiar and predictable ingredients (lettuce, tomatoes, cucumbers, carrots) along with more novel choices, such as sliced daikon radishes, jicama, fresh spinach, colorful pepper slices, fresh sliced mushrooms, pea pods, green cauliflower and sliced summer squash.

▲ **PASTA SALAD:** This recipe is a great summertime dish. Offer some or all of the following ingredients: chilled cooked whole grain pasta in at least two different shapes, chopped or grated vegetables (e.g., carrots, broccoli, cauliflower, sweet peppers, jicama, zucchini), grated Parmesan or Romano cheese, sliced olives, avocado chunks and mushrooms. Once students have assembled their salad, instruct them to mix it with Italian dressing or vinaigrette.

▲ **PERFECTLY PERSONAL PIZZA:** Students learn to create their own pizza recipe, perfect for a quick mini-meal or snack. Using whole grain English muffins or bagel halves as the base, spread with tomato sauce, sprinkle on spices, add toppings and sprinkle with grated part-skim mozzarella cheese. Examples of toppings include chopped onions, pepper rings, sliced black or green olives, mushroom pieces, broccoli or cauliflower florets, tomato slices, chopped turkey or ham and lean hamburger or ground turkey

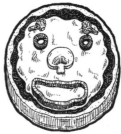

that has been browned and drained. Try spices such as oregano, garlic, basil, thyme, parsley or marjoram.

To cook pizzas, bake at 400 degrees for 8–10 minutes or broil for 3–5 minutes.

Calculating Nutrients and Physical Activity
(ADVANCED ACTIVITY)

Intermediate students interested in calculating their precise intake of calories, protein, fat, calcium, iron or other nutrients can use an online program or software designed for nutrient analysis. There are also tools that are designed to help track physical activity and fitness goals.

▲ The USDA sponsored *SuperTracker* is an online tool based on the 2010 Dietary Guidelines for Americans and the *MyPlate* food guide. The *SuperTracker* can help plan, analyze and track diet and physical activity. You can look up the nutritional value of individual foods, find recommendations for what and how much you should eat, compare your food choices to these recommendations and assess personal physical activity level. The program can be accessed at the choosemyplate.gov site.

▲ There are several programs available for purchase that analyze dietary intake. Most programs also compare intake to a standard recommendation based on age, gender and activity level. Data is usually presented in a variety of ways, including graphically. Although most programs are geared for students at the secondary level, many fourth and fifth graders possess the skills needed to use these programs. Many of these software packages are also designed to analyze the nutrient content of individual recipes. (See Appendix B, audiovisual resources, for catalogs that carry nutrient analysis software.)

▲ Is there an app for that? As technology continues to change and evolve, there will be a growing number of nutrition and physical activity "apps" designed for smart phones, touchscreen tablets and other electronic devices and games. Be sure to preview and screen these programs to make sure they are well designed and appropriate for children.

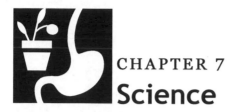

CHAPTER 7
Science

"Thank you for coming. I didn't know that (for) every pound we gain your heart has to beat an extra mile." —Mark

When my daughter was a first grader, she approached me about project ideas for her school science fair. I naturally thought of all the possibilities that related to food and nutrition science. The idea that sparked her interest the most was to survey her classmates and analyze their eating habits. By the time we finished this project, she had gained skills in a variety of subject areas. She developed a simple questionnaire that her classmates used to record their diets for one day, analyzed and compared their daily diets with the *Food Guide Pyramid* (the recommended food guide at the time) and presented her data graphically, using her best art skills to design, color and display her work.

Because nutrition is a science, the prospects for science activities are limitless. This chapter presents learning ideas in three areas: food in the body, the study of plants as food and how kids can use the scientific method to conduct nutrition research.

Food in the Body

Nutrition is the science of how the body uses food. Even young children can gain an appreciation of how food is broken down and used inside the body. The food we eat goes through five stages of processing: **digestion**, **absorption**, **circulation**, **metabolism** and **excretion**. Simple explanations with engaging experiments and activities will bring these concepts to life.

TASTE AND SMELL

Our experience with food starts with our **nose** and **tongue**. The sensation of taste is actually a combination of smelling the food and using the taste buds on our tongues. While it was once believed that we use different areas of our tongues to taste different sensations including salty, sweet, bitter or sour, scientists now believe that we actually can detect most types of taste with most of our taste buds. In other words, the idea of the "tongue map" is an outdated concept that is not backed by science.

Scientists have also discovered an additional taste sensation known as umami (pronounced oo-mommy) which is thought to be the savory or meat-like taste found in the chemical glutamate. Examples of foods with the umami taste include meats, mushrooms, aged cheeses and soy sauce.

ACTIVITY

▲ At snack or mealtime, instruct children to take a bite of one food and describe how it tastes. Next, have them hold their noses and take a bite of the same food. Ask them to describe the taste of the food and how it changed. Discuss how the sense of smell plays a part in detecting the flavor of foods. That is why the sense of taste is diminished when we are suffering from colds.

DIGESTION

Digestion is the process of breaking food down into millions of tiny pieces. Beginning in the **mouth** and ending in the toilet, food covers a route about 25 feet long, all inside the body! After the mouth, food travels to the **stomach** by way of a tube known as the **esophagus**. Most of the "action" of digestion occurs in the **small intestine**, a coiled-up organ that completes digestion and transfers nutrients through its walls to the blood stream. This so-called "small" intestine would stretch around 20 feet long if it were uncoiled. In the **large intestine** (larger around, but much shorter in length than the small intestine), water is added to waste products, making a paste that can be excreted.

While food is broken down somewhat by chewing and grinding, most digestion takes place by body chemicals. Chemicals known as **enzymes** break down food in the mouth, stomach and small intestine. Other chemicals include **acid** in the stomach and **bile** (which helps break down fat), which is released into the intestine by the gall bladder.

The Digestive System

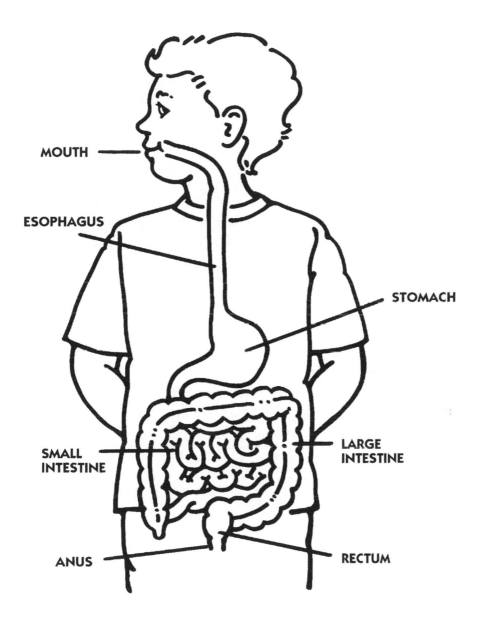

MOUTH

ESOPHAGUS

STOMACH

SMALL INTESTINE

LARGE INTESTINE

ANUS

RECTUM

ACTIVITIES

▲ Working in pairs, have students trace an image of their body onto large sheets of paper. Enlarge and reproduce or project page 101 on your classroom projector. Ask students to draw and label the parts of the digestive tract on their life-sized silhouettes.

▭ How can the digestive tract measure more than 20 feet long in a child who is just four feet tall? How could that be? Using a tape measure and string, have students measure 25 feet of string. Using their life-sized body silhouette, ask them to "fit" the digestive tract into the one they just drew, affixing it with glue if they wish.

You Will Need:

♦ Projected image of page 101

♦ Large sheets of paper

♦ Tape Measure

♦ String (25 feet per child)

For tasting Activity:

♦ Sugar-free crackers

♦ Napkins

▲ Even as we are enjoying the taste of food in our mouths, digestion is beginning. As the teeth grind and crush the food, an enzyme in the saliva begins breaking down carbohydrates into sugar. To demonstrate this concept, pass out small pieces of a saltine or a similar bland sugar-free cracker. (See Appendix A before you conduct a tasting activity). Read the label, pointing out that the crackers do not contain added sugars. Ask students to hold the cracker on their tongues without chewing or swallowing. What do they taste? After a few minutes, ask students whether the taste of the cracker has changed. Elicit possible explanations for this happening. Explain that the sweet taste means a chemical called an **enzyme** in their saliva has digested the starch to sugar.

▦ Who was the first scientist to understand that body chemicals, not just mechanical action, are responsible for digestion? In 1822, an ambitious army doctor named Dr. William Beaumont was able to conduct digestion experiments on a living man! When fur trader Alexis St. Martin was shot in the stomach, he survived despite slim odds. But a small hole into his stomach never successfully healed, allowing Dr. Beaumont to conduct a multitude of digestive experiments and withdraw stomach acid for study. This fascinating story is told in the children's book, *Dr. Beaumont and the Man with the Hole in His Stomach*, by Sam and Beryl Epstein

(Coward, McCann & Geoghegan, 1978). Read this book to the class or encourage intermediate students (third through fifth grade) to read and report on it. Note: The book is out of print but can be located in many libraries or purchased through online booksellers.

▲ The most slowly digested nutrient is fat. That is why a greasy meal can leave a person feeling stuffed for hours. One reason is that fat travels through the digestive system in big droplets or globules. When fat encounters the dark liquid **bile** in the small intestine, it is broken down into small droplets. Bile acts as an **emulsifier**, a substance that can break fats into small globules that will mix with water.

You Will Need:
♦ Clear glass
♦ Water
♦ Vegetable Oil
♦ Egg
♦ Tablespoon
♦ Spoon

Using water, liquid vegetable oil and a raw egg yolk, students can observe how bile breaks down fat during digestion. An egg yolk contains the emulsifier lecithin. (Lecithin is often added to salad dressings and other processed foods because it breaks up the fat particles, resulting in a smooth product.) In a clear glass, mix 1 cup of water and 2 tablespoons of oil. What happens? Try stirring the mixture vigorously. Does the fat break down? Next, add the egg yolk to the mixture and stir. What happens to the fat droplets? This reaction is similar to how bile breaks down fat in the small intestine. (Incidentally, egg yolks do not work as emulsifiers in the body since they are changed by both cooking and stomach acid before they reach the small intestine.)

ABSORPTION

After food is digested into small particles, it must somehow move from the digestive tract to the rest of the body. That movement into the bloodstream is called **absorption** and happens mainly in the small intestine.

The small intestine is made up of millions of fingerlike projections called **villi**. The villi are covered with a hair-like brush that traps the nutrients. The nutrients are then passed through the villi into tiny blood vessels called **capillaries** which eventually empty into the body's major blood vessels.

ACTIVITIES

▲ To explain the concept of absorption visually, use a carpet sample to illustrate the surface of the small intestine. Each yarn fiber sticking out of the carpet is like a villus, ready to absorb nutrients and pass them into the bloodstream.

You Will Need:

♦ A carpet sample

Books for young readers that explore digestion include What *Happens to a Hamburger*, by Paul Showers (HarperCollins Juvenile Books, 2001) and *Burp! The Most Interesting Book You'll Ever Read About Eating*, by Diane Swanson (Kids Can Press, 2001).

CIRCULATION

How do nutrients find their way up to your nose and down to your toes? Every cell of the body requires a continuous supply of energy from nutrients and oxygen from the air we breathe. Oxygen and nutrients are transported to cells by **arteries**, while **veins** carry carbon dioxide and waste products out of the cells. This network of blood vessels, including the small, web-like, connecting vessels known as **capillaries**, makes up the circulatory system. The **circulatory system** relies on a very important pump, the **heart**, to continually move blood throughout the body.

ACTIVITIES

The hard-working heart needs good care to work at its best. Eating a balanced diet, participating in at least 60 minutes of physical activity each day and controlling stress are all important heart-healthy habits to develop at a young age. Chapter 11 includes information and activities about the role diet and exercise play in keeping the heart healthy. The American Heart Association has a wide array of curricula designed to teach children about the heart and how to keep it healthy. Visit www.heart.org and click on the link for educators.

METABOLISM

Once nutrients finally make their way to the billions of tiny cells that make up the body, they are used to supply the building blocks for energy, healing, maintenance and growth. Each cell of the body is like a tiny factory, taking the raw materials of nutrition and producing energy or growth and replacement parts. At any given moment, the cells of an active child are busy supplying energy to run at recess, creating new cells to make bones and muscles bigger, sending sugar to the working brain, and producing skin cells to heal a scraped knee.

Fortunately, the body does all these things without conscious effort. The only thing a healthy child really needs to think about is eating a diet that supplies the necessary raw materials.

ACTIVITIES

▲ What is hunger? It is the body's message to the brain that more nutrients are needed for growth, maintenance, repair and energy. By the time hunger sets in, the body's energy stores are running low and the ability to focus on tasks becomes difficult. To illustrate this point, ask children to respond to their hunger in other ways than eating: by reading, doing math problems, taking a walk, etc. If possible, delay their scheduled snack break or lunch period by 30 minutes in order to carry out this experiment. NOTE: Ask permission from parents before conducting this activity. This is not an appropriate activity for children with certain medical conditions such as diabetes or hypoglycemia.

Ask the children how they felt while doing other activities when hungry. Were they able to concentrate? How was their energy level? Their mood? Discuss the role that nutrition plays in learning. Point out that kids who skip meals, especially breakfast, often don't learn as well as kids who eat regular meals.

Benefits of Breakfast

Breakfast contributes to health and development and also fuels brain cells for learning. An optimal breakfast is made up of nutrient-rich foods and includes a source of protein (from protein foods or low-fat dairy), a serving of whole grains, and either a fruit or vegetable. Research shows that when kids eat breakfast, they:

♦ Are more likely to get the nutrients they need to get through the morning. Breakfast eaters have higher daily intakes of fiber, calcium, vitamin A, vitamin C, riboflavin, zinc and iron compared to kids who skip breakfast.
♦ Have higher test scores, miss less school and are tardy less often.
♦ Are more likely to focus, concentrate, solve problems and learn.
♦ Behave better in the classroom.
♦ May have an easier time achieving a healthy weight.

⊟ ⊞ Ask students if they know what the word "breakfast" means (break the fast). Explain that a fast is a period of time without food. Ask students to calculate how many hours their body normally "fasts" from suppertime to breakfast.

On the board, write the sentence "Breakfast is the most important meal of the day." Ask students to write or tell whether this statement is true and why or why not. Encourage them to write about their own experiences with breakfast, including where and what they usually eat.

EXCRETION

The final stop for food is the excretion of waste products. Even the most nutritious food has parts that cannot be digested and absorbed into the body, e.g. fiber. After food leaves the **small intestine**, it enters the **large intestine** where water is added to form a paste that can be easily excreted. Other nutrient waste products are filtered through the **kidneys** and excreted through the urine (breakdown products of protein metabolism and salt, among others).

ACTIVITY

As part of your weekly vocabulary and spelling words, assign intermediate students some or all of the bolded words from the *Food in the Body* section:

Absorption	Enzymes	Mouth
Arteries	Esophagus	Nose
Bile	Excretion	Small intestine
Capillaries	Heart	Stomach
Circulation	Kidneys	Tongue
Digestion	Large Intestine	Veins
Emulsifier	Metabolism	Villi

Plants as Food

Studying and growing edible plants is a wonderful way to reinforce nutrition and introduce children to scientific concepts and processes. Observation, prediction and data collection are skills gained by applying science to gardening. A "growing" classroom or home can be as simple as a few seeds planted in a milk carton or as elaborate as a greenhouse or large outdoor school or community garden.

Encourage young botanists to keep a journal as they study and grow edible plants.

> **Check this out:**
> Patten, E. & Lyons, K. (2003). *Healthy foods from healthy soils: a hands-on resource for educators.* Gardner, Me: Tilbury House Publishers.
> This resource combines ecology, science and nutrition into a comprehensive and easy-to-use guide. Throughout the guide, "Spokesworm" Annelida gives you the dirt on soil, gardening, composting and more.

PHOTOSYNTHESIS

A miracle really, life as we know it starts in the leaves of a plant. Using energy from the sun, carbon dioxide and water, chlorophyll-containing cells in green plants manufacture carbohydrate. Plants comprise the first link of the food chain, providing food energy for other living organisms, including people.

ACTIVITY

▲ To observe the effects of photosynthesis, start with a green potted plant. Instruct children to observe, draw and record how the plant looks. Place it in a dark closet. Continue to water regularly but do not expose to light. Every two days, bring the plant out briefly to allow children to observe and record the changes. How does the plant change? Ask children to draw a conclusion about the effect light has on plants. Explain that when light is removed, photosynthesis cannot occur and the plant is unable to manufacture food.

> **You Will Need:**
> ♦ A green potted plant

GERMINATION

Even when dormant for a period of years, seeds will sprout when given the right conditions of warmth and moisture. This process is called germination.

ACTIVITY

▲ To watch germination in action, place dry beans in a clear glass jar containing a moistened sponge and place on a windowsill. The sponge will keep the seeds moist and hold them against the side of the jar where they are visible. Ask children to carefully record or draw the germination process in their plant journals, including any predictions they make about the process or how long it will take. (And later, notes on whether their predictions came true and why or why not.)

Ask if any of the seeds sprouted "upside down" or "sideways" (the answer should be "No"). Elicit from the students how seeds know to sprout "right side up." (ANSWER: Seeds respond to gravity by sprouting root down, stem and leaves up. This concept is known as phototropism.)

Caution: This is not an eating activity! Discard the sprouts once the project is completed. Commercial as well as home-grown sprouts pose a risk for foodborne illness. In most reported cases of illness linked to sprouts, salmonella and E. coli. were present in the seeds. For more information, visit foodsafety.gov.

GROWING VEGETABLES

Organic planting mix, empty milk cartons, and a sunny window (or grow light) will suffice for young gardeners just starting out. For classes who wish to garden on a larger scale, there are a number of programs and grants available designed to assist schools in setting up a school-wide, comprehensive gardening curriculum. Before you embark on a school garden, be sure to check out the resources at right.

School gardening resources

♦ healthymeals.nal.usda.gov/hsmrs/garden/
A comprehensive site with links on how to start and maintain a school garden and connect the garden with the classroom

♦ www.edibleschoolyard.org
The edible schoolyard project

♦ www.GardenABCs.com
A resource rich sharing site for school gardening

♦ www.kidsgardening.com
Grant information and much more from the National Gardening Association

♦ www.lifelab.org
Comprehensive site with an emphasis on gardening and environmental education

The activities below are designed to spark interest and encourage children to involve their families in planting gardens at home. Most can be carried out with minimal time and expense.

ACTIVITIES

▲ Radishes are a great vegetable for the beginning gardener. Many varieties germinate in 4–7 days and are ready to eat in 25–28 days. First, fill cleaned containers or half-pint milk cartons with planting mix. Read the seed packet instructions to find out the planting depth (usually 1/4 inch). Ask students to think of ways they can accurately measure the soil to arrive at the correct planting depth (a ruler or marked stick will work). Next, have students place four to five seeds in the soil (apart from each other), cover lightly and gently water. To maximize drainage, poke a small hole in the bottom of the carton and place on a lid or in a tray.

> **You Will Need:**
> ♦ Radish seeds
> ♦ Small containers or clean half-pint milk cartons
> ♦ Organic planting mix

Encourage students to describe the planting process in their journals. Ask children to predict when their seeds will germinate and how the seedlings will look when they first sprout. Every day, students can check on their plants and record any observations or changes. Keep plants moist but avoid overwatering.

Once the seedlings sprout, encourage students to make daily or weekly measurements and/or predictions about the growth and record them in their plant journals. Results can be presented in a variety of ways — through drawings, tables or graphs, for instance.

The radishes should be thinned to two plants per carton. They are ready to pick and eat when the roots become round and begin to pop up out of the soil. After harvesting, weigh the radishes and record that in the plant journals. Wash, slice and taste the radishes or use them to make one of the radish garnishes described in Chapter 10.

▲ A great springtime gardening activity is to "start a salad." Students can then take their seedlings home and plant them in small garden patches or in large pots placed on their decks or patios.

Materials to start a salad include an empty paperboard egg carton, organic planting mix and a variety of salad seeds. If possible, take the class on a field trip to a garden center or nursery to choose seeds for this project. Examples of salad greens include spinach, arugula, kale, watercress and lettuce varieties such as romaine, oakleaf, butternut and redleaf. Fill egg carton compartments with planting mix and plant seeds according to package directions. When they have reached a height of 2 inches, send them home with a note to parents, encouraging them to transplant the plants outside or into a larger container. For easy transplanting, cut apart the compartments of the carton, poke a hole in the bottom of each compartment, and place it in the soil, carton and all.

You Will Need:

♦ Paperboard egg cartons

♦ A variety of "salad" seeds (see text)

♦ Organic planting mix

Encourage children to monitor the progress of their "salad" and record their findings in their plant journals.

▲ Just like all living things, plants have a lifecycle. Growing lettuce can make a fascinating study of the lifecycle of a plant. As a class project, plant and grow lettuce in a large container in the classroom. Observe and record the progress of the plants and taste the lettuce when it reaches maturity. Allow at least one of the plants to "go to seed," a process where the lettuce will produce long shoots with flowers. Eventually the flowers will form small seed pods. (This process, from start to finish, takes a few months.) Start all over again by harvesting and planting the seeds — a perpetual experiment!

You Will Need:

♦ Large plant container

♦ Lettuce seeds

♦ Planting mix

Ask students why plants "go to seed" and why harvesting seems to prolong the process. Discuss the ways other fruits and vegetables produce seeds. Ask students to bring in examples from home (e.g., avocado pit, cantaloupe or melon seeds) and experiment with planting.

Children's Books about Gardening

♦ Cherry, L. (2003). *How groundhog's garden grew*. New York: Blue Sky Press.

♦ Coy, J. & Fisher, C. (2009). *Two old potatoes and me*. New York: Dragonfly Books.

♦ Ehlert, L. (1987). *Growing vegetable soup*. San Diego: Harcourt Brace Jovanovich.

♦ Gibbons, G. (2008). *The vegetables we eat*. New York: Holiday House.

♦ Grigsby, S. (2010). *In the garden with Doctor Carver*. Chicago, Ill: Albert Whitman.

♦ Grigsby, S. (2012). *First peas to the table: how Thomas Jefferson inspired a school garden*. Chicago, Ill: Albert Whitman.

♦ Milway, K. & Daigneault, S. (2010). *The good garden: how one family went from hunger to having enough*. Toronto: Kids Can Press.

♦ Nagro, A. (2011). *Our super garden: learning the power of healthy eating, by eating what we grow*. United States: Dancing Rhinoceros Press.

PARTS OF PLANTS WE EAT

The vegetables we commonly eat comprise a wide variety of plant parts. The activities below allow young botanists to classify, observe and eat various parts of plants.

ACTIVITIES

▲ Explain that vegetables can be classified according to the edible part of the plant. The six general categories are roots (including tubers and bulbs), stems, leaves, fruits, flowers and seeds. The classification of a vegetable as the "fruit" part of the plant can be tricky. Explain that a "fruit" refers to the edible part that grows from a flower and contains seeds on the inside. The "fruits" that lack significant sweetness are generally classified as vegetables. It's interesting to note that there are differences in the way nutritionists and botanists (plant scientists) classify certain vegetables. Brainstorm examples of vegetables in each category:

Roots: carrot, beet, radish, turnip (potatoes are technically tubers while onions are bulbs)

Stems: celery, asparagus

Leaves: lettuce, spinach, kale, cabbage

Fruits: tomato, cucumber, eggplant, squash, pepper, pumpkin

Flowers: broccoli, cauliflower, artichoke

Seeds: corn, pea, green bean

▲ Take a field trip to a grocery market, farmers' market or produce farm. Encourage children to take note of the variety of produce they see. Upon return to the classroom, make a list of the observed vegetables and name the part of the plant each comprises.

Before you conduct the following food activities, review Appendix A, "Guidelines for Safe Classroom Cooking." Make sure you communicate with parents and inquire about any food allergies, intolerances or medical conditions that will influence the foods that you can use in this activity.

▲ Bring a variety of vegetables into the classroom for observation and tasting. Include less common varieties, including daikon radishes, broccoli-cauliflower hybrid, Brussels sprouts, bok choy and kale. Provide hand-held microscopes that students can use to examine the vegetables.

You Will Need:

- A variety of vegetables
- Hand-held microscopes
- Cutting board and knife
- Plastic gloves
- Small plates or napkins
- Clean hands

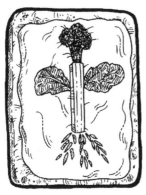

⊠ Make "plant-part art" for a snack. You will need large, flat crackers; nut butter or low-fat cream cheese; broccoli florets; celery sticks; lettuce leaves torn into small pieces and shredded carrots. Students will first spread crackers lightly with either cream cheese or nut butter. Next, they will create a plant or garden design using shredded carrots for roots, celery sticks for stems, lettuce for leaves and broccoli for flowers. This is also a fun and effective way to encourage children to taste vegetables.

You Will Need:

- Large, flat crackers
- Nut butter or low-fat cream cheese
- Broccoli florets
- Celery sticks
- Lettuce leaves
- Shredded carrots
- Plates or napkins
- Clean work area
- Plastic gloves
- Clean hands

Using Science to Answer Food & Nutrition Questions

Children can practice using the scientific method and also learn answers to food and nutrition questions at school or home. The scientific method involves formulating a **question**, developing a **hypothesis**, coming up with a **method** or experiment to test the hypothesis, evaluating the **results** and forming a **conclusion**. The hypothetical examples below illustrate how kids can apply this method to food and nutrition research. Students should also be encouraged to take the results of their experiments and use them to make recommendations for change.

Even very young scientists need to understand a few rules before setting up research experiments. It is important to get the permission of everyone involved, including cafeteria staff, administrators, students and parents. Individuals should not be pressured or forced into participating and individual results should always be kept confidential.

GARBAGE AS SCIENTIFIC EVIDENCE

Kids can monitor the cafeteria garbage to answer questions about what kids eat or throw away at lunchtime. The example below outlines one possibility for an experiment. Working in groups, students can come up with other ways of monitoring diets and influencing cafeteria choices by studying plate-waste.

Question: Which fruit do second grade students eat more of: fresh grapes or canned pears?

Hypothesis: Second grade students will eat more fresh grapes than canned pears.

Experiment: Empty lunch trays will be checked on two different days, including one day when fresh grapes are on the menu and one day when canned pears are on the menu. Students will stand by the area where second graders return their dirty trays and record whether the fruit was eaten, partly eaten or not eaten. The first twenty second graders who return their dirty trays will be studied each day.

Results: On the day fresh grapes were served, 12 of the 20 second graders ate the entire serving, 5 ate part of their grapes and 3 students did not eat any grapes. On the day canned pears were served, 6 of the 20 second graders ate the entire serving, 4 ate part of their pears and 10 did not eat any pears.

Conclusion/Recommendation: Hypothesis confirmed. Second graders prefer fresh grapes to canned pears. They ate more and wasted less on the day that fresh grapes were offered. The school lunch menu should offer fresh grapes more often and canned pears less often. Better yet, kids should get a choice of two or more fruits every day in order to eliminate waste and improve nutrition.

NOTE: Depending on the level of the students, the results can be manipulated mathematically, using graphs to plot raw results, or converting to percentages and presenting the data in a table or graph.

FINDING OUT ABOUT OTHER PEOPLE'S DIETS

Is it nosy to ask people what they eat? Maybe, but the government does it all the time when they conduct surveys of Americans' eating habits. Conducting nutrition surveys is a fun and informative way to learn about and compare the diets of different groups of people. Surveys can be descriptive, telling about the diet of a certain group of people (e.g., 8-year-old soccer players). Or a survey can be comparative, contrasting the difference in eating habits between two groups of people (e.g., soccer players versus piano players). The example below is a comparative study.

Question: Who eats or drinks more low-fat dairy products: third grade girls or third grade boys?

Hypothesis: Third grade boys consume more low-fat dairy products than third grade girls do.

Experiment: Design a simple checklist that includes the following foods: 1 cup fat-free milk, 1 cup 1% milk, 1 cup low-fat yogurt, 1 cup fat-free yogurt and 1½ ounce low-fat cheese. Ask third grade students to check off each serving of low-fat dairy products that they eat or drink for two days.

Remind them to pay attention to the serving size, making one check mark for each amount listed. (For example, if they eat 3 ounces of cheese at one sitting, that's two check marks.) Do not tell them that you are comparing girls to boys — they may make a contest out of it, which will bias the results. Instead, explain that they should eat and drink just as they normally do. Collect the surveys after two days.

Results: Fifteen girls and ten boys completed the survey. For the two days, the fifteen girls consumed 60 servings of low-fat dairy foods. The boys consumed 50 servings of low-fat dairy foods in two days. Using averages, the girls ate an average of 4 servings each in the two-day period (60 servings divided by 15 girls). The boys ate an average of 5 servings each in the two-day period (50 divided by 10 boys).

Conclusion: Hypothesis confirmed. Third grade boys ate an average of 2.5 servings of low-fat dairy products each day while third grade girls ate an average of 2 servings of low-fat dairy products each day.

MORE IDEAS

Once their minds are set in motion, students will enjoy using science to answer other food and nutrition questions. Encourage children to work cooperatively when planning and conducting their research. Perhaps the best gratification is that their projects can help initiate change in nutrition practices or policies.

Below is a brief list of other possibilities for nutrition research.

A study reported in the *Journal of the American Dietetic Association* showed that students ate more at lunch when they had recess before lunch. Test this hypothesis in your school, comparing two similar classrooms that have different recess/lunch schedules.

Working with the school cafeteria manager, set up taste tests with students for new nutritious foods offered by food manufacturers.

▲ Do a comparison study between kids who bring their lunches from home and those who get lunch at school.

▲ Nutrients that are commonly in short supply in the diets of pre-adolescents include iron, calcium, vitamin E and folate. Analyze and identify foods in the cafeteria that are good sources of these nutrients and create a poster to display the information in the cafeteria. A useful online resource for nutrient analysis is the food composition database from the USDA. You can access it online at www.ars.usda.gov/ba/bhnrc/ndl

▲ If candy or cookie sales are a common school fundraiser, offer to study whether selling nutritious snacks (whole grain crackers, nuts, dried fruit, trail mix, apple slices, string cheese etc.) can be just as profitable.

▲ Poll teachers in the school to see how many teach nutrition in their classrooms.

▲ Design a study to test whether breakfast cereals with toys in the packages contain more sugar than cereals without toys.

Table 7-1

What About Organic Foods?

Certified organic foods are now widely available in most mainstream grocery stores. Grown without the use of pesticides, synthetic fertilizers, or genetically modified organisms, organic farming employs green principles of agricultural production. Animals that produce meat, poultry, eggs and dairy products are raised without the use of antibiotics or growth hormones.

Research studies have shown that eating organic foods significantly lowers the pesticide exposure in children. In one study, children who changed from a conventional to a totally organic diet had undetectable levels of pesticide byproducts in their urine after just a few days.[1]

Encourage intermediate students to obtain accurate information and use critical thinking skills to make informed decisions about complex issues such as organic foods. It is also important to reassure children that all fruits and vegetables are nutritious and that many people cannot afford an all-organic diet. To learn more about the issues surrounding organic foods and agriculture, check out the following resources.

♦ www.ams.usda.gov/nop
   USDA Agricultural Marketing Service National Organic Program

♦ www.ewg.org/foodnews
   Environmental Working Group, publisher of the Shopper's Guide to Pesticides in Produce™

1. Lu, C., Toepel, K., Irish, R., Fenske, R., Barr, D., & Bravo, R. (2006). Organic diets significantly lower children's dietary exposure to organophosphorus pesticides. Environmental Health Perspectives 114(2): 260-3.

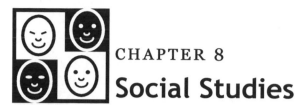

CHAPTER 8

Social Studies

"Your visit was FUN! Now I like vegetables more. My Mom and Grandma make Korean food — they make exotic animals! Since I was small my Grandma wanted to teach me it. Now they were impressed (by) what I learned." —Tara

My childhood was filled with interesting food experiences, though I seldom appreciated their richness at the time. My grandmother of German descent prepared the most marvelous pastries, homemade noodles and Kraut Bieroch, a hamburger-cabbage mixture wrapped in delicious bread dough. My father, the son of a Greek immigrant, practiced his heritage by cooking wonderful Greek dishes. The week before Dad made Kapama', a chicken-based tomato dish served with ziti pasta and cheese, the whole house smelled of drying goat cheese, usually feta or kefalotyri.

Most notably, I grew up on a farm where we had a large garden (almost a mini-farm in itself), fresh milk, fresh eggs from a neighbor and food cooked mostly from scratch. Of course, I didn't realize at the time that our rural Nebraskan lifestyle would be viewed by today's standards as trendy, green and sustainable. We were locavores and didn't even know it!

A major goal of this chapter is for children to appreciate how dietary habits and traditions vary between individuals and cultures. Children will learn to identify and evaluate their own dietary customs and also explore the food habits of people from other cultures.

A unit on corn stresses the role that this grain played in history and the continuing importance of corn in modern-day America.

Finally, guidance is given for students interested in studying the problem of hunger in their community. Exploring issues surrounding hunger creates awareness and spurs students to take action to help those who lack access to nutritious food.

Identifying Individual Food Culture

Everyone eats, of course, but the what, where, when and even how of eating vary tremendously. Children don't need to go far to appreciate the diversity in food traditions. Even within a single classroom, children can discover great variety in family food habits and customs. Besides differences in ethnic origin and religion, families make choices based on personal preference and convenience. The activities below will help students identify their own traditions and perhaps start a few new ones.

ACTIVITIES

Identifying Food Customs: Ask students to think about and complete the questions listed in Worksheet 8-1 concerning their food environments. Encourage them to design and share projects that explain their answers in a creative way. For instance, students can write and illustrate stories about their families' meals, design and perform a skit, develop videos of their families' mealtime traditions or create drawings, paintings or posters that depict their families at mealtime.

▲ **Carrying the Message Home:** Be sure that children share their work and ideas with their families. Invite family members to visit, share recipes and describe their own childhood food experiences. Consider hosting a potluck or a recipe exchange that features food favorites from each family. (Check local school and health department regulations before planning a potluck.)

Blending Food Traditions: What happens when people from different cultures develop relationships and eat together? The book, *How My Parents Learned to Eat*, by Ina R. Friedman (Houghton Mifflin, 1987), explores how a Japanese woman and an American sailor overcome insecurities about their different eating customs.

In the "Everybody Cooks..." series by author Norah Dooley, neighbors of different ethnicities and backgrounds use the same staple food in many ways. Dooley's titles include *Everybody Cooks Rice* (Houghton Mifflin, 1996), *Everybody Bakes Bread* (Carolrhoda Books, 1996), *Everybody*

Name_____

Identifying Your Food Customs

Everyone grows up with different food customs. The following questions will help you to identify your family's unique food culture.

1. Name and describe all the people in your family.

2. Does your family eat together? How often? Which meals?

3. Who decides what your family eats? Who shops? Who cooks? Who cleans up the mess?

4. Are there foods that your family especially likes to eat? Name and describe them.

5. What is your favorite food? Who makes this food? How often?

6. Arc there special foods that your family eats on holidays or during religious celebrations?

7. Does your family sometimes eat foods that originated in another country? Name and describe.

8. Describe a meal or celebration with food that was especially fun or meaningful (e.g. Thanksgiving dinner, Bar Mitzvah, Birthday celebration).

9. Is there anything about your family's eating habits that you wish you could change? Describe the changes.

10. Fill in the blank: one tradition that I would like my family to begin is to _____. (Examples: Eat breakfast together on Sundays; Allow the kids to plan the menu once a week; Turn the TV off at dinnertime; Eat in a restaurant every other week; Try foods from other countries once a month).

May duplicate for educational use

Serves Soup (First Avenue Editions, 2004) and *Everybody Brings Noodles* (First Avenue Editions, 2005). All books in the series include recipes.

Another book that explores differing perceptions about food traditions is *Family Dinner*, by Jane Cutler (iUniverse, 2011). Geared for the intermediate reader, this is the story of how a modern-day family who doesn't "do dinner" reacts to the efforts of visiting Great-Uncle Benson who insists "you can't have a family without a family dinner."

More children's books with multicultural food themes are described below.

Multicultural Children's Books with Food Themes

♦ Browne, E. (1999). *Handa's surprise.* Cambridge, Mass: Candlewick Press. For a description, see page 67.

♦ Diakite, B. (1999). *The Hatseller and the Monkeys.* New York: Scholastic Press. For a description, see page 71.

♦ Gershator, D. (1998). *Bread is for eating.* New York: H. Holt. All phases of bread production are presented with colorful characters and illustrations in a multicultural format. The phrase "El pan es para comer" (translation: Bread is for eating) is repeated throughout, with the complete song included at the end. This heart-warming story is presented in both Spanish and English.

♦ Grigsby, S. (2010). *In the garden with Doctor Carver.* Chicago, Ill: Albert Whitman. For a description, see page 68.

♦ Hester, D. (2007). *Grandma Lena's big ol' turnip.* Morton Grove, Ill: Albert Whitman & Co. In a retelling of a Russian folktale, Grandma Lena grows a gigantic turnip in her garden. The book features a multi-generational African-American family who work together to harvest the turnip and then enjoy the results when Grandma Lena cooks a soul food feast.

♦ Lin, G. (1999). *The ugly vegetables.* Watertown, MA: Charlesbridge. This is a tale about a little girl who thinks her mother's Chinese vegetable garden is ugly, especially compared to the neighbor's flower gardens. She changes her mind after her mother makes a delicious soup from the vegetables. Recipe included. Companion activities are also included at the author's website located at www.gracelin.com.

♦ Mora, P. (2007). *Yum! mmmm! qué rico! Americas' sproutings.* New York: Lee & Low Books. Fourteen plant foods which are indigenous to the Americas are explored through information about the food's origin and history, Haiku, fun facts and colorful illustrations.

Food Cultures around the World

Many different types and combinations of foods can be used to nourish the body. This becomes evident when studying various cultures and noting the differences in early native diets. But perhaps most interesting is the striking similarity in the nutritional composition of many native diets throughout the world.

Since the dawn of agriculture — roughly 10,000 years ago — people around the world have relied on a dietary staple rich in complex carbohydrate, most commonly a grain such as rice, corn, wheat, barley, sorghum, oats, buckwheat or millet. In some cultures, the primary staple is a starchy root such as potatoes, yams, cassava (tapioca) or taro. According to anthropologist Sidney W. Mintz, these carbohydrate sources provide more than half of the world's calories.

In addition to this dietary core of complex carbohydrate, virtually all cultures include a high-protein legume such as peas, beans, peanuts, chickpeas (garbanzo beans) or lentils. Food historian Ken Albala, author of *Beans: A History* (Berg, 2007), writes:

> *"Nearly every place on earth has its own bean species, and each was paired with a grain staple in ways that literally made civilization possible. Think of beans and corn in Mexico, soy and rice in China, or wheat and pulses such as fava beans, chickpeas and lentils in the Middle East. Lesser known, though equally important are black-eyed peas with yams or millet in Africa."*

In reference to this pairing of grains/carbohydrates with legumes, Mintz noted, "This almost universal pattern in the diet of farmers is hard to explain; but whatever the reasons, it has been nutritively advantageous for our species."

Examples cited by Dr. Mintz include red beans and corn tortillas in Mexico; bean curd, mung beans and rice in Japan; wheaten bread accompanied by hummus (chickpea paste) in the Middle East; and, in Caribbean countries, rice or millet paired with red or black beans.

From a nutritional point of view, the pairing of grains with legumes forms a "complete" protein that contains the full array of essential amino acids (the building blocks of protein) needed for growth, cell replacement, formation of important proteins such as enzymes and hormones and repair of body cells and tissues.

ACTIVITIES

▲ **Learning about Dietary Staples:** Explain to children the concept of "dietary staple," that is, a food that makes up a large piece of the diet, usually a carbohydrate such as a grain or a starchy root. Ask them why it is important to have a food rich in carbohydrate as a staple. Ask if they recall the body's first and most important need, nutritionally speaking. (ANSWER: Energy — see page 45 for a description.)

Discuss how cultures around the world have developed diets that are nutritionally similar, featuring grains or starchy roots for carbohydrate and beans, lentils or nuts for protein. Elicit reasons why different cultures living far apart managed to develop similar diets. Point out that early agrarians needed carbohydrates as a staple because their lifestyle as physical laborers required a great deal of energy.

> **Check this out:**
> D'Aluisio, F. & Menzel, P. (2008). *What the world eats.* Berkeley, Calif: Tricycle Press. The author and photographer are cultural geographers who traveled the world, documenting the food habits of twenty-five families in twenty-one countries. Perfect as a classroom reference, this book features fascinating stories and full-colored photographs, including a display of a week's worth of food and groceries for each family.

Ask students to think and list examples of ethnic diets that feature a combination of grains and plant protein. Common examples include tortillas and beans from Mexico, lima beans and corn (a mixture known as succotash) from American Indians, and rice and bean curd (tofu) in Asian cultures.

Because of advances in transportation and the global exchange of commodities, people throughout the world now consume a diet comprised of a wide variety of foods. In developed countries such as the United States, there is a greater reliance on animal foods for protein, calcium and other nutrients.

It's hard to characterize the "American diet," since the diversity of people that comprise our culture has resulted in an interesting blend of different flavors and cuisines. Ask students to discuss how they would describe the American diet to someone from another culture.

Name_____

What's Your Staple Carbohydrate?

A staple refers to the food or foods that make up the biggest portion of a diet. Most early civilizations had a very limited diet that almost always centered on a staple which was high in carbohydrate.

Find out if you have a staple carbohydrate by keeping a record of what you eat for one to three days (using more than one day will give a more accurate picture of your diet). Record how many servings of carbohydrate-rich foods you eat in the proper spaces below.

NOTE: The standard serving size is listed beside each food. Be sure to take this size into account when counting your servings (e.g. If you eat 1 cup of pasta, that is equal to 2 servings).

WHEAT:
___Pasta (1 serving = ½ cup) (e.g. macaroni, spaghetti, noodles)
___Wheat Flakes Cereal (1 serving = 1 cup)
___Bread (1 serving = 1 slice)
___Bagel (1 serving = ½ bagel)
___Hamburger Bun (1 serving = ½ bun)
___English Muffin (1 serving = ½ muffin)
___Flour Tortilla (1 serving = 10" tortilla)
___Orzo (1 serving = ½ cup)   ___Couscous (1 serving = ½ cup)

OATS:
___Oatmeal (1 serving = ½ cup cooked)   ___Dry Oats Cereal (1 serving = 1 cup)

RICE:
___Cooked Rice (1 serving = ½ cup)   ___Crispy Rice Cereal (1 serving = 1 cup)

CORN:
___Cooked Corn (1 serving = ½ cup)   ___Corn Tortilla (1 serving = 10" tortilla)
___Corn Flakes (1 serving = 1 cup)

POTATOES:
___Baked Potato (1 serving = 1 medium)   ___Mashed Potatoes (1 serving = ½ cup)
___French Fries (1 serving = 12 medium) ___Sweet Potatoes (1 serving = ½ cup)

OTHERS:
___Barley (1 serving = ½ cup)   ___Millet (1 serving = ½ cup)
___Amaranth (1 serving = ½ cup)   ___ Plantain (1 serving = ½ cup)
___Quinoa (1 serving = ½ cup)   ___ _____

After you complete this worksheet, answer the following questions:

1. Do you have one staple carbohydrate or do you rely on lots of different foods to supply your body with carbohydrates?

2. Why do you think people in early civilizations ate high carbohydrate diets?

3. According to the *MyPlate* guide, how many servings (ounces) of grains should you aim for in your daily food plan? (You can find out at www.choosemyplate.gov)

May duplicate for educational use

▲ **What's Your Staple Carbohydrate?** In this activity, students will keep a diet record for one to three days in order to identify if their diets have a staple grain or starchy root (tuber). Enlarge and reproduce the "What's Your Staple Carbohydrate?" Worksheet 8-2 on page 125 and pass it out to students. Students will count the number of servings from each grain or starch and record it on the worksheet. After they have completed the activity, ask them to draw conclusions and share with the class. While some may be able to identify one particular staple carbohydrate, many will notice that they eat a wide variety of grains and roots. Ask them how they think their diets differ from that of their early ancestors.

In terms of nutrition, the *MyPlate* food guide recommends fewer servings of grains than in past U.S. food guides. This reflects the growing issue of obesity and also the recognition that most modern-day Americans are not engaged in heavy physical labor or exercise.

▲ **Identifying Grains:** Collect grain samples, including common varieties (rice, oats, corn, wheat), a few that are lesser known (barley, millet, quinoa, triticale, amaranth, teff, etc.) and as many of the corresponding flour or meal products as possible. Set up a center where students can identify and label the grain and flour samples. Provide a mortar and pestle so students can experiment with grinding the grain kernels.

You Will Need:

♦ Grain samples (see text for ideas)

♦ Variety of flours and corn meal

♦ Mortar and pestle

▲ **World Food Map:** Display a large classroom-sized map of the world, labeling it "World Food Map." Assign students the task of researching one country to determine a common food or group of foods eaten in this country. (This can be an extension of an assigned report on a particular country.) They can find out this information by talking to people from this country; researching online sources, ethnic cookbooks, almanacs and encyclopedias in the library; or calling or visiting restaurants that feature food from their assigned countries.

The Multicultural Cookbook for Students, by Carole Lisa Albyn and Lois Sinaiko Webb (Greenwood Press, 2009) is an excellent resource for adults and advanced students, complete with interesting and authentic recipes.

Recommended resources for younger readers include *The Kids' Multicultural Cookbook: Food & Fun Around the World*, by Deanna F. Cook (Williamson Publishing, 2008), *Around the World Cookbook* by Abigail Johnson Dodge (DK Publishing, 2008) and *The Coming to America Cookbook* by Joan D'Amico and Karen Eich Drummond (Wiley, 2005).

The following examples taken from the *Children's Britannica* illustrate one source of information that students can access. The school librarian can offer help on locating library and online resources for this research.

JAPAN: "Japanese-style meals include very little meat, butter and cheese. The chief food is rice served in a bowl and eaten with chopsticks. A great deal of fish is eaten, sometimes raw, and other foods include pickled vegetables, bamboo shoots, bean-curd soup, sweet potatoes and fruit."

RUSSIA: "The chief item of Russian meals continues to be bread, which is usually of the "black" (actually very dark brown) kind. Other traditional dishes are shchi, which is a cabbage soup, and kasha, a grain porridge. Specialties of Russian cooking are pirozhki (little meat pies), blini (pancakes), borscht (beetroot soup) and various forms of sour milk and cream."

ITALY: "The main meal, usually at midday, often begins with soup, which may contain rice, pasta or greens. This is followed by meat or fish, cheese and fruit. In parts of the Po valley, polenta, or cooked corn, is common and a lot of barley and chestnuts are eaten."

Give each child a 3" x 5" notecard on which to describe the assigned country's diet. They can do this in a variety of ways. They can write down the foods commonly eaten, draw a picture of the typical foods or an example of a meal, glue small pieces of dried food (rice, corn, beans, etc.) to the card or create their own representation of the country's diet.

Allow each child to give a short report on what he or she learned about the assigned country's diet. With the help of the students, find the countries on the World Food Map and tack the notecards on the designated countries.

Going Further: Ask students to find and share a recipe for a food commonly eaten in their assigned countries.

▲ Plan a class party or celebration that includes an ethnic theme and food. Examples include African dishes at a Kwanzaa celebration, Mexican food or Cinco de Mayo, or a potlatch to celebrate Native American culture.

Diversity in the School Cafeteria: Invite the school nutrition manager into the classroom to discuss how he or she plans menus that meet the needs and preferences of different ethnic groups in the school. For instance, some ethnic groups have a high incidence of lactose intolerance, which limits their ability to digest milk products. Other groups cannot eat pork or beef because of religious restrictions. Ask if there are ways that the school nutrition program accommodates these and other groups.

▲ Work with the school nutrition manager to plan menus and events that emphasize the ethnic diversity of the school community. Each month, a different grade or classroom could be assigned to develop a promotion for one ethnic group, complete with decorations, music, clothing or costumes, skits or dances and, of course, food.

> **Check this out:**
> Lauber, P., & Manders, J. (2009).
> *What You Never Knew About Fingers, Forks and Chopsticks.*
> New York: Simon & Schuster Books for Young Readers.
> Starting with cavemen and moving throughout history, this delightful and humorous book covers the history of eating utensils and customs.

▲ Offer to share recipes, food customs and traditions of various cultures with the nutrition manager. Suggest ways that the cafeteria can integrate these foods into the monthly menu, perhaps by offering a rotating "ethnic bar" on a regular basis.

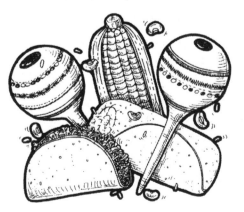

🧩📺 A Corn Unit

A grain with historical significance, the study of corn makes an ideal cross-curricular unit. Besides discussing the nutritional contribution of corn, the history, modern-day uses and experience by different cultures make a fascinating study.

BOOKS

Children will enjoy learning about the history, cultivation and many uses of corn in the books *Corn*, by Gail Gibbons (Holiday House, 2008), *Corn is Maize: The Gift of the Indians*, by Aliki (HarperCollins, 1986) and *From Kernel to Corncob*, by Ellen Weiss (Children's Press, 2008).

A well done and engaging reference for adults who are preparing to teach this unit is *The Story of Corn* by Betty Fussell (University of New Mexico Press, 2004).

HISTORY

Corn, also called maize, is indigenous to the Americas, comprising the staple food of many early Native American tribes. Corn spread to the rest of the world only after Columbus landed in the West Indies and obtained corn from the natives he named the "Indians." The earliest American settlers would have starved if the natives had not given them corn to cook, eat and grow. It was so valuable that the settlers used it instead of money to trade with the Indians for food and furs.

Most of the corn used by Native Americans was dried and ground into cornmeal using a flat stone called a metate, a job that was difficult and laborious. Today, powerful machinery in modern-day mills grinds and processes corn.

Eventually, the production and selling of corn became a way of life for many people who settled in what is now known as the "corn belt" of America (which includes Illinois, Indiana, Iowa, Kansas, Minnesota, Missouri, Nebraska, Ohio and South Dakota).

ACTIVITIES

Obtain several ears of field (also known as dent) corn from a local mill or farmer. Set up centers where children can explore various aspects of corn:

▲ First, children can remove the husks and silk from the ears, a process known as husking. Ask students if they can name the state known as the "cornhusker state" (ANSWER: Nebraska). Next, they can shell the kernels from the cob for use in the following activities. Ask children if anyone knows the name of the machine that picks and shells large fields of corn (ANSWER: A combine).

Experiment with grinding the kernels. Provide a mortar and pestle, instructing students to grind one or two kernels at a time. (It's a difficult task.) Ask students to write or tell a story about how it must have felt to grind corn by hand, all day long for many days, like the Native Americans once did. (Some remote tribes still grind corn and other grains by hand.)

Native Americans and early settlers used all parts of the corn, including the husks and cobs. Husks were used to make dolls and art, braided into masks and stuffed into mattresses. Cobs were burned for fuel and made into corn-cob pipes. Ask students to brainstorm unique uses for cobs, husks and silk. Encourage children to use them in creative art projects.

Using small containers or empty half-pint milk cartons, organic planting mix and fish emulsion, plant three to four corn kernels in each carton. (Native Americans used fish to fertilize the soil when they planted corn.) Observe and record the sprouting and growth of the corn plants. See Chapter 7 for more on growing plants.

USES AND VARIETIES

It would be difficult to make it through one day without experiencing a food or product made from corn. In the average supermarket, there are thousands of food items that contain corn. Besides the obvious — cornmeal, corn flakes, corn chips, popcorn and grits — there are a multitude of products that contain corn syrup, corn oil and cornstarch.

The biggest use for the corn grown in America is animal feed. Corn is also used to make many nonfood items, ranging from tires and gasoline to glue, soap, medicines, plastics, cloth and many other products.

Although there are many varieties of corn, the four most common are two field varieties (dent and flint), sweet corn and popcorn. Field corn is used for animal feed, ground into meal and made into corn syrup, oil and starch. Sweet corn is a softer, sweeter type of corn that is eaten fresh on the cob, frozen and canned. Popcorn is eaten primarily as a snack food. Specialty corns gaining popularity include blue and white varieties, which are often made into gourmet corn chips.

ACTIVITIES

▲ Send students on a "corn hunt," either at home or at a local supermarket, checking ingredient labels to find products that contain some form of corn. Divide the products into two lists, one that includes foods that are primarily made from corn (e.g., corn nuts, corn tortillas, ready-to-eat corn cereals, hominy) and those that have corn-based additives such as corn syrup, dextrose or corn starch (e.g., ketchup, pudding, soft drinks).

"CORNY" FOODS	
Main Ingredients	Corn Additives
Corn Flakes	Pudding
Corn Tortilla	Pancake Syrup
Hominy	Soda Pop
Popcorn	BBQ Sauce
Corn Oil	Gravy

Count how many items on the monthly school lunch menu that contain some type of corn.

▲ Invite a corn farmer to speak to the class. Better yet, take a field trip to his or her farm. Other possibilities include visiting a mill that grinds corn or a factory that processes corn.

▲ As a class, have a cooking/tasting party of corn recipes that represent various cultures. Examples include corn tortillas (Mexico), corn bread (Native American) and ugali (cornmeal porridge native to Kenya). Good sources for authentic recipes include *The Multicultural Cookbook for Students*, by Albyn and Webb (Greenwood Press, 2009) and *Foods of the Southwest Indian Nations: Traditional & Contemporary Native American Recipes*, by Lois Ellen Frank (Ten Speed Press, 2002).

NUTRITION

While corn is rich in complex carbohydrates and a good source of plant protein, it is far from a complete or perfect food. In the early 1900s, people in the United States who relied primarily on corn as their dietary staple often developed the disease pellagra, caused by a deficiency of the B vitamin niacin. The disease had also been described in Italy and Spain as early as the 1700s. Interestingly enough, Indian and Mexican cultures who first soaked their corn in lye or lime avoided pellagra. (Scientists now understand that the lye reacts with corn to release the amino acid tryptophan, which the body can then transform into niacin.)

Using corn (or nearly any single food, for that matter) as an exclusive food inevitably leads to nutrient deficiencies. That is why *MyPlate* is based on the premise that a variety of foods are needed for optimal nutrition.

Is corn a grain or a vegetable? The answer depends on if you ask a botanist (answer: grain) or a nutritionist (answer: it depends). In the *MyPlate* food guide, fresh, frozen or canned sweet corn is classified as a starchy vegetable while products made from field corn such as corn tortillas, cornbread, cornmeal, grits and polenta are classified as grains.

To maximize nutrition, look for whole grain corn tortillas, cornmeal, cereals and other products that list whole corn as the first ingredient. Popcorn is always a whole grain, since the entire kernel is "popped." The key to healthy popcorn is to avoid products with a lot of added fat and/or sugar. It is cheap and easy to make air-popped popcorn and add just a small amount of butter or other flavorings.

ACTIVITIES

▲ Students who enjoy research can study and report on the disease pellagra, and how the U.S. Bureau of Public Health and doctors in the early 1900s finally solved the mystery of why people who ate mostly corn often developed this fatal disease. (A similar story to research and report is how a diet of polished rice led to the thiamin deficiency disease beriberi.)

▲ **Going Further:** Students can note the nutritional contribution that various grains make to the diet through careful label reading. Suggest that students visit online retail sites that sell a variety of different flours (e.g. www.bobsredmill.com) and check the *Nutrition Facts* labels of whole-wheat flour, corn flour and oat flour to compare the levels of fiber, protein and iron in each product. Ask students to discuss which grain contributes the most nutrients to the diet.

Helping Those in Need

Millions of Americans with limited resources go hungry each day. Faced with scarce pantries and empty refrigerators, many rely on community food banks and soup kitchens to make it through each month. Since food banks rely mostly on donations, the foods distributed through emergency food agencies are not always the most nutritious. Emergency food providers often fall short of dairy, fruit, vegetable and lean protein items.

All ages are touched by this problem, including an estimated 16.2 million U.S. children who live in food-insecure households. Hunger in America often goes unnoticed because few develop the telltale signs of severe malnutrition such as the wasted bodies and bloated bellies seen in drought- and war-torn developing countries. While few American children are on the brink of starvation, many are unable to perform or learn well due to marginal nutrition and transient hunger. Virtually every community throughout America is touched by the problems of poverty and hunger.

Children can become involved by learning, participating and offering solutions to the hunger problem in their community.

ACTIVITIES

▲ Invite a staff member from the local food bank, soup kitchen or other community agency to speak about the problem of hunger. Ask the guest to describe the extent and impact of hunger, dispel myths about people who are hungry, describe efforts underway to solve the problem and brainstorm with children ways they can contribute to the solution.

▲ Sponsor a schoolwide "nutrition drive" for the hungry, emphasizing donations of healthful nonperishable foods. Brainstorm lists of canned and dry foods that fit the guidelines of *MyPlate*. Using the blank *MyPlate* on page 52 as a model, create a drawing with examples of nutritious nonperishable donations. Send this list, along with information on the nutrition drive, home with all students in the school. Be sure to include information on how people who lack enough nourishing food can find help in the community.

Table 8-1

Suggestions for Nutrition Drive Donations	
FOOD GROUP	**Examples of Nutritious Non-Perishable Foods**
Grains	low sugar whole grain breakfast cereals, oatmeal, packaged dry pasta, brown rice, quinoa, couscous, popcorn, whole grain pancake mix, baby rice cereal
Vegetables	canned vegetables, canned low-sodium vegetable and tomato juice, spaghetti or pizza sauce, baby food vegetables
Fruits	dried fruit, canned fruit (in its own juice), canned, boxed or bottled 100% fruit juice, applesauce (with no added sugar), baby food fruit
Dairy	low-fat milk in aseptic packaging, nonfat dried milk powder, soy beverage in aseptic packaging, dried grated Parmesan cheese
Protein Foods	canned meats such as chicken, tuna, salmon, sardines; canned or dried beans, split peas and lentils; peanut butter almond butter, packaged nuts, canned soups, stews and chili, baby food meats
Oils and "Extras"	Canola oil, olive oil, canned olives, fruit jam

▲ To promote the nutrition drive to the school and community, plan activities that increase awareness of hunger issues. Students can create and perform a skit on hunger, make posters and flyers, decorate food barrels or promote the drive through local supermarkets.

You Will Need:

♦ Pots for planting

♦ Organic Planting Mix

♦ Variety of flower, fruit and vegetable seeds

Enterprising young gardeners can raise money and awareness for hunger by selling vegetable and flower starts in the Spring. Start plants such as tomatoes, peppers, melons or flowers in small pots indoors approximately eight weeks before the sale. (See Chapter 7 for information on growing plants.) Tie the sale in with another event, perhaps a Mother's Day tea, music program, field day or other Spring school event. Working in groups, students can set up and decorate their plant stand, write an "advertisement" to send home to parents and take turns staffing the stand. Students will gain practice in running a business and develop math skills by changing and counting money.

If the school has a community garden, consider donating fresh vegetables to agencies that serve those who are hungry or homeless. Children may also want to plant and grow vegetables over the summer in their home gardens. Encourage donations of extra garden produce to agencies that serve the hungry.

Check this out:
Milway, K. & Daigneault, S. (2010). *The good garden: how one family went from hunger to having enough.* Toronto: Kids Can Press. This is a moving story that explores global hunger and food insecurity from the perspective of one poor farm family in Honduras. A valuable and interactive companion website to this book is located at www.thegoodgarden.org.

CHAPTER 9

Performing Arts

"Thank you for the radish spinners,
They were just a treat.
Thank you for the pickle fans,
They were sour but good to eat.
Thank you for the orange peeled rose,
That looks pretty while standing in a pose." —Sweeta

Collaborating with a middle school drama teacher proved to be a gratifying experience. We worked with eighth grade drama students in the production of a nutrition play for elementary students. The idea was to motivate the younger children to try more healthful foods. I lent the nutrition expertise while Portland drama teacher Adele White worked her magic, inspiring the students to create and perform a delightful 20 minute play. Using the costumed dog characters Sheggy Good-Grub (who eats from all five food groups) and Sickly Spot (who subsists on extras such as candy, soft drinks and fried snacks), they enacted the consequences of nutrition choices in a play they titled *"Sickly or Successful: You Decide."*

The students performed the play for area elementary schools, leading the audience in stretching exercises during intermission. The event was a huge success — the younger children were mesmerized during the play and nearly knocked Spot over (who transformed from "Sickly" to "Successful") after the play.

The biggest surprise of all was the effect the process had on the actors. While eighth graders are not always known for making healthy food choices, the students took an interest in nutrition and began asking me questions about their personal health and eating habits. (Granted, I did see cookies back stage a time or two.) They even ate and enjoyed the healthy vegetable-loaded pizza that I served at the stage party.

Through the process of acting, role playing and teaching others, students are able to internalize nutrition knowledge, making them more inclined to practice good eating habits. Studies conducted in Minnesota verify that performing arts are an effective way to create awareness and impart knowledge about health and nutrition to elementary students.

Chapter four (pages 58-59) gives guidelines on setting up classroom dramatic play areas for children in the early grades. Presented here are ideas on how to incorporate nutrition into performing art exercises and events. The children — so naturally dramatic and wonderfully creative — will inspire the best ideas. Please allow it!

Role Playing

Role playing in small familiar groups is a great exercise that allows children to creatively and cooperatively solve problems. Use realistic, familiar scenarios that kids face when making decisions about food. Stress that there are no right or wrong answers but instead, the goal is to practice making choices and to explore the consequences of those choices. Use the ideas listed in Table 9-1 or create your own.

Creating Food and Nutrition Ads

Creating their own food advertisements helps children to understand the motive behind the messages that blitz their everyday lives. After reviewing the advertising techniques described below, set up activities that allow students to practice identifying these techniques in real ads. The final step is to use these methods to create positive ads touting healthful foods, balanced nutrition, positive body image, exercise or other health-promoting habits.

TECHNIQUES USED IN ADVERTISING

Advertisers use a variety of means to influence and persuade kids, many of which are cleverly disguised as games or promotions. The list below describes some of the ways advertisers commonly market products to children.

▲ **Popular Characters or Celebrities:** Advertisers often appeal to the emotional attachment children have for an athlete, musician, animated character or television/movie star. Popular characters are licensed to sell a multitude of products — clothing, books, puzzles, toys and also foods such as

Table 9-1

What Would You Do?

Working in small groups, encourage children to develop and act out solutions to the following scenarios.

♦ Your friend thinks she is too fat so she decides to go on a diet that she found in one of her mom's magazines. She wants you to go on the diet, too. How would you handle this situation?

♦ After school, you always feel so hungry. When your mom's not looking, you grab a bunch of cookies and go outside to play. Later, you don't feel hungry for supper. What would you do next time you're hungry after school?

♦ You like it when your Dad packs fruit, vegetable sticks and other healthful foods in your lunch. But the kids at school tease you about eating healthful foods, calling you "veggie head." How would you solve this problem?

♦ Your friend says that a "Giggles" candy bar is healthy because the commercial on TV showed kids with lots of energy after they ate Giggles. He is now convinced that Giggles will give him energy, too. What would you tell him?

♦ On school mornings, you would rather sleep longer and skip breakfast. You really aren't that hungry when you first wake up, anyway. But lately, you have noticed that after morning recess, you have a headache, your stomach growls and it's hard to do your work. How would you solve this problem?

♦ You always have to rush to make it to afternoon soccer practice on time. You usually grab a can of pop and a package of potato chips to eat on the way. The problem is, your stomach often starts hurting in the middle of practice, especially if you have to run a lot. What do you think is causing your stomach aches? What changes could you make to solve this problem?

♦ Your best friend is a picky eater who rarely eats from the five food groups. You have noticed that he looks pale and tired and gets sick a lot. What could you do to help your friend?

♦ Your mom is a health-food nut. She is forever bringing home strange-looking vegetables with even stranger-sounding names, things like bok choy, kohlrabi and rutabaga! Worse yet, she expects you to eat them. You flatly refuse, saying you will not try anything that looks or sounds strange. Is there a better way to deal with this situation?

♦ Your big sister is pretty and popular but all she ever eats are salads and diet soft drinks. She says most other foods are "fattening." Is she right? What would you say to her?

♦ Your parents went out for the evening, leaving you with a teenage babysitter. She says you can have whatever you want for dinner, even candy! What foods would you choose?

May duplicate for educational use

cereal, candy and fried snack foods. Likewise, celebrities are paid millions of dollars in endorsements to peddle sugary drinks, fast food and empty calorie snacks to kids.

▲ **Constant Exposure:** Marketing has become very sophisticated, barraging children with nonstop messages. Besides television commercials, children may also be exposed to in-school promotions and company-sponsored curricula, kids' clubs with special promotions and glossy magazines, online advergames and product placements in movies and sporting events.

▲ **Exaggerated Health Benefits:** The nutrition or health benefits of foods marketed to children are often greatly exaggerated in advertisements. Products that contain little fruit are praised by dancing fruit characters or shown with images of real fruit. Candy bars are played up for their ability to "energize." Highly sweetened cereals claim to be "part of a nutritious breakfast." Sweetened non-juice beverages that are essentially liquid sugar are fortified with 100% of the daily value of vitamin C in an attempt to convince kids and parents that the beverage has some nutritionally redeeming value.

▲ **Free Toys:** Many food products appeal to children because they feature free toys or other mail-order giveaways. Fast food kids' meals are a notorious offender, enticing kids with cheap plastic toys while instilling a taste for French fries and burgers. Toy offers are also often placed strategically in grocery store aisles where kids will be sure to notice them.

▲ **Disguised Ads:** Advertisements in children's magazines are often cleverly disguised as comic strips, games or puzzles. Kids often think they are just another feature in the magazine. Websites and apps for mobile devices are filled with appealing "advergames" that promote foods or products to kids.

▲ **Wearable Advertisements:** Many children are unknowingly walking ads for products. Shirts, jackets, backpacks, water bottles, sports jerseys and other everyday items often sport highly visible company logos.

Name_____

Discovering the Motive Behind the Message

This worksheet will help you to analyze how advertising and marketing influence the foods you buy (or ask your parents to buy). Use the checklist below to decide which methods are used to promote this product.

Food Advertised:_____

1. Describe the advertisement (e.g. magazine ad, TV or radio commercial, online advergame, name or logo on a product, etc).

2. Check the categories below that apply to this food advertisement:

____Popular Characters or Celebrities
Does the ad feature popular sports figures, celebrities or animated characters?

____Constant Exposure
Is the product marketed in many different ways? Do you often see this product promoted on the internet, television, radio, billboards, magazines, clothing, etc.?

____Exaggerated Health Benefits
Do the ads for this product try to make you think that the food is nutritious or a good source of energy?

____Disguised Ads
Does this advertisement look like it could be part of a website, school assignment or magazine? Is it presented in cartoon, puzzle or story form so it doesn't look like an ad?

____Wearable Advertisements
Is the company name or logo on something you can wear or carry such as a shirt, jacket, backpack or water bottle?

3. Did this advertisement make you more likely to buy the product? Explain.

4. Do you think the claims made by this ad are true? Why or why not?

May duplicate for educational use

ACTIVITIES

▲ Ask children to bring in examples of advertising that use one of the techniques described above, including online links to commercials. Set up a center where students can identify and label the advertising technique, using Worksheet 9-1 as a guide.

▲ For homework, ask students to watch at least one hour of children's programming on Saturday morning (excluding public television). Using Worksheet 9-2, have them keep track of how many commercials are for food. Based on what they know about nutrition, ask them to estimate whether the foods advertised are healthful (i.e., one of the five food groups, reasonable in fat and sugar content). Ask them to note if there were any Public Service Announcements (PSAs) that promoted healthful eating.

▲ Contrast the goals of the advertiser with those of the consumer. Explain that companies are in business to make money and advertising is an important way to inform and also persuade people to purchase their products. Advertising also supports television programs, radio, magazines, many websites, social media sites and apps for mobile devices. Discuss or debate the merits of advertising, posing questions like "What responsibilities do advertisers have?" or "Should advertising to kids be banned?" or "Should companies who advertise concern themselves with children's health?"

> **Check this out:**
> Burstein, J. (2008). *Big fat lies: advertising tricks.* New York: Crabtree Publishing Co.
> This children's book from Slim Goodbody takes an inside look at the world of advertising.

For information on how to write to food companies or television networks, refer to the suggested writing activities aimed at the young nutrition advocate on pages 79-80.

CREATING A COMMERCIAL

Once children are familiar with the techniques used by advertisers, they can use this knowledge to create and perform their own 1- to 2-minute commercial for a nutritious diet, specific food, healthy body image or other healthful habit like exercise. Working in small groups, children can follow the steps below to create and perform their ad for the class, parents or

Name_____

Taking a Look at Saturday Morning Food Ads

To complete this activity, you will watch at least one hour of Saturday morning programming on a commercial network, such as ABC, CBS, NBC, Fox or Nickelodeon. Once you decide on the channel, do not switch networks until you have finished this assignment.

Network Watched: _____

Date watched: _____

What time did you start watching? _____

What time did you stop watching? _____

Every time you see a food commercial, make a tally mark beside the category below that best describes the food advertised.

_____ Candy
_____ Soft drinks
_____ Sweetened beverages (not 100% juice)
_____ Sweetened cereal
_____ Corn chips, potato chips or other fried snacks
_____ Cakes, cookies or pastries
_____ Sweetened fruit snacks
_____ Other sweetened foods

Food Groups:
_____ Grains (e.g. low-sugar cereals, waffles, pasta, rice)
_____ Fruits (fresh, frozen or canned, 100% fruit juices)
_____ Vegetables (fresh, frozen or canned, vegetable juices)
_____ Protein (e.g. meat, chicken, seafood, beans, eggs, peanut butter)
_____ Dairy (e.g. milk, cheese, yogurt, soy beverage)

Others:
_____ Combination Meals (e.g. children's frozen dinners)
_____ Fast food restaurants
_____ Public Service Announcements promoting good nutrition

_____ _____

Questions:

1. How many total food advertisements did you see during the time you watched?

2. How many of these were for foods that you consider nutritious?

3. How many of these were for foods that are not the most nutritious?

4. Do you think there should be more advertisements for healthy foods on television? Why or why not?

May duplicate for educational use

other students. In some school systems, students may even have the opportunity to record their commercial as a Public Service Announcement (PSA) for local television or radio stations.

▲ **Brainstorm:** As a group, decide which healthful food or idea about good eating you want to sell. Examples include a breakfast promotion, healthful snacking, a specific fruit or vegetable, whole grain foods for energy, dairy foods for bone health, protein for a growing body, water as the best beverage to quench thirst or the importance of reading *Nutrition Facts* labels.

▲ **Create a Storyboard:** Working together, students will decide how to convince other kids to buy their products or take their advice. They will create a storyboard, which is the script for a commercial that contains both words and pictures. The storyboard tells all the specifics of the commercial, including details about music, actors, props, etc.

▲ **Assign Roles:** Once the storyboard is done, the group will decide who is responsible for each role. Students will decide who will direct, act, be in charge of music and design props for the commercial.

▲ **Design Props or Costumes:** Students can create simple costumes or props on their own or enlist the help of parent volunteers.

▲ **Rehearse:** Students should practice the commercial until they feel it is polished enough to perform in front of others. They may also need to make minor adjustments to the storyboard or adjust the length of the commercial (it should not exceed two minutes).

▲ **Perform the Commercial:** Students can perform their ads for the class, other classes, the whole school during lunchtime or as part of a parent program. Videotaping the commercial gives students the chance to critique and enjoy their work.

▲ **Evaluate the Campaign:** Real advertisers want to know if their commercials work. Suggest students develop and pass out a simple questionnaire which asks the audience whether they are more inclined to try the food or suggestions just advertised.

Producing Skits and Plays

The possibilities are endless when it comes to developing skits and plays. Children can make and manipulate puppets, dress up as food characters or act as celebrity chefs who host cooking shows. Kids who enjoy music and art can find or write songs and design sets and props. The ideas in this section are meant to spark kids' creativity.

A helpful resource is the video *Janey Junkfood's Fresh Adventure* from the theater company FOODPLAY. An Emmy award winner, the program uses rap music, juggling, splashy graphics and dynamic young actors to communicate important nutrition messages. A companion book is described on page 74. Find out more at www.foodplay.com.

> **Check this out:**
> Registered dietitian Jill Jayne is the highly entertaining **Rockstar Nutritionist!** She performs live nutrition and health themed rock 'n roll concerts for kids. Visit her website www.notetohealth.com to learn about her shows and order her original nutrition rock music.

SKITS

A skit is a short play with a simple message. Skits range from impromptu classroom exercises (such as the role-playing activity above) to productions that are elaborately planned and rehearsed.

At school, quick skits (15 minutes or less) can be used to promote an event or send an important message, as the examples below illustrate.

Work with the school cafeteria manager to promote a new food or menu. Perform a short skit in the cafeteria during each lunch period.

Develop and perform a skit about hunger and its consequences to promote a nutrition drive for the needy (see page 134).

Demonstrate the link between nutrition and exercise in a skit that promotes a school fun run, walk, field day or other school wide athletic event.

To promote environmental awareness, plan a skit that emphasizes nutritious foods with minimal packaging. Demonstrate how certain food scraps can be recycled to make compost. Students will enjoy acting as worms, demonstrating the breakdown of food to soil.

PLAYS/VIDEO PRODUCTIONS

A play or video production is often longer than a skit, and usually involves more preparation, backdrops, costumes, props and music. Some ideas:

▲ **MyPlate Play:** The name of the latest food guide, *MyPlate,* conjures up images of the classic "Who's on first?" dialogue. For example:

> Student one: "Have you seen MyPlate?"
> Student two: "No, I haven't seen your plate."
> Student one: "No, it's not your plate, it's MyPlate. Have you seen it?"
> Student two: "Like I said, I haven't seen your plate."
> Student one: "No, it's MyPlate!"

Students can create an original play about the *MyPlate* food guide that resolves this dialogue.

▲ **The Evening News:** Build a play or video production around the theme of a news broadcast. Feature a late breaking segment about how "label reading before eating alerts kids to possible nutrition dangers," human interest stories about kids who changed their lives through a more healthful diet, cooking segments, an opinion-based commentary on food advertising and a live, on-the-scene coverage of the school cafeteria in operation.

▲ **Seasonal/Holiday Plays:** Put a nutrition twist on seasonal or holiday productions. Examples include "Goblins Who Gobble Good Goodies," "The Diet of the Pilgrims," "Frosty the Snowman Melts off Pounds," "How to Be Sweet without Sweets on Valentine's Day," "Why St. Patrick Likes His Greens," "Why Bunnies Don't Eat Chocolate" or "Nutrition and Your Teeth: Advice from the Tooth Fairy."

PUPPETRY

Children enjoy manipulating puppets and inventing stories. A classroom puppet area or theater is a good place for students to express feelings and create dialog. To encourage scenes about nutrition and fitness, include food props, puppet-sized jump ropes or personified food puppets. Kids enjoy making their own puppets, whether out of felt, paper bags, construction paper (finger puppets) or other materials.

Children can create a traveling puppet play on health and nutrition that they can perform for younger children.

Teachers or nutrition professionals can also learn to use puppets effectively. It doesn't take a great deal of skill to tell a story with a puppet or two. The amazing thing is that children will automatically be drawn to the puppet on your hand, even though they realize the words come from you. Speaking through puppets gives adults a chance to express ideas and knowledge in a new, refreshing way. Kids respond differently to a message from a puppet, too. (That's why puppets are often used to promote open communication with children who have been abused or have emotional disorders.)

Creativity Tips

Whether producing a commercial, play, video, skit or puppet show, the following ideas are fun ways to communicate good-food messages.

▲ Interject humor by using food as edible props. Use a banana for a phone, carrot or cucumber for a conductor's baton or fruit as juggling balls. An even more comical approach is for the characters to eat the props as they use them!

▲ A nice addition to a production is the use of poems about food or silly nutrition songs set to common tunes.

▲ Puppets can be used as props within a play or video production. Food puppets can hover over a character's head, playing the role of the "conscience," which tries to convince kids why they should be eaten. A puppet show can also serve as an effective "play within a play," or as a television show or commercial set within a play.

> **Check this out:**
> Musician Jay Mankita writes and performs songs for kids about animals, ecology, and healthy food. He has made his 10 song album about fruits and vegetables available as a free download at eat-like-a-rainbow.bandcamp.com

▲ Kids can play the part of life-sized food models. To help children "feel" the part, have a tasting party using real foods. As children taste apples, asparagus, French bread or farmer's cheese, have them imagine how the texture, appearance and flavor would transfer into a character role. An orange, for instance, may decide to act in a very sour manner, the cheese wedge might portray a mellow character or the grapes may decide to act very sweet.

▲ Build on the writing activities in chapter 5 by suggesting that students role play the stories and descriptions that they write. See *Putting a Nutrition Twist on Fairy Tales* on page 76 and *Descriptive Writing* on page 78.

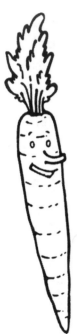

Create a "Madame Food-sauds" Wax Museum

Create a museum of food using the children as the "waxed" fruits and vegetables. Assign each child a specific fruit or vegetable and instruct them to research interesting facts about their produce, including how it grows, major nutrients, the best way to prepare it and maybe even a short recipe. A great resource for this information is the "More Matters" website from Produce for Better Health, located at www.fruitsandveggiesmorematters.org.

Children can put together costumes that represent their fruits or vegetables. To create the effect of a wax museum, have them stand perfectly still with paper "on" switches on the floor near where they are standing. To activate the wax figure, visitors will step on the switch. The fruit or vegetable then comes to life and begins the presentation on how it grows, why it is good to eat, etc. This is a great presentation to do for parents' night at school.

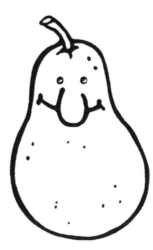

A Classroom Breakfast Song

Breakfast helps to start your brain.
Fruit or veggie, milk, whole grain.

When you wake up, eat some food.
You will feel strong and good.

Every morning, start out right.
Eating breakfast keeps you bright.

Sing to the tune of "Twinkle, Twinkle, Little Star" in primary class-rooms or have older students develop an upbeat rap version. Encourage students to create additional verses about the link between breakfast and learning. See page 105 for more about the importance of breakfast.

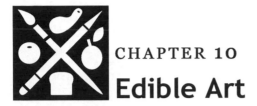

CHAPTER 10

Edible Art

"Thank you for showing us how to make those fruit sculptures. Last night I asked my mom to buy some oranges and she did. I tried to make a rose but I didn't do it but I did better." —Krystal

More than mere cooks, many chefs are artists in their own right. Instead of paints and canvas or chisels and bronze, their medium is food and their tools are kitchen gadgets and knives. Like artists who make oceanside sand sculptures, the art created by chefs is transient, but beautiful nonetheless.

These edible art ideas will capture the imagination of children as they delight in playing with their food. Some of the activities are easy while others require more practice. They are all designed with safety in mind — they can be completed using plastic serrated knives and other tools that are safe when properly handled.

Aside from the artistic merits of their work, children will also enjoy eating their creations. I have found that children are more willing to try new foods when they are involved in preparation and cooking activities.

> **Check this out:**
> Elffers, J. & Freymann, S. (2006). *Fast food.* New York: Arthur A. Levine Books.
> Elffers and Freymann are masters of transforming fresh produce into an art form. They have a number of food art books with full colored photos including *Food Play* and *How are you peeling? Fast Food* is my personal favorite because it depicts fruit and vegetable sculptures engaged in various modes of transportation, including physical activities such as walking, bicycling, ice skating, skateboarding and more.

Before you conduct food activities with children, review Appendix A, "Guidelines for Safe Classroom Cooking." Make sure you communicate with parents and inquire about any food allergies, intolerances or medical conditions that will influence the foods that you can offer.

Note: Most of the food activities in this chapter are open ended and flexibile in terms of the type and amounts of specific ingredients. Therefore, only the recipes that include ingredients in precise quantities include nutritional information.

Zigzag Fruits

INGREDIENTS/SUPPLIES:

- 1 piece of fruit per child (Oranges, lemons, grapefruits, firm kiwifruit or large strawberries work well.)

- plastic ridged or semi-ridged knives, plates

- clean work surface and hands

DIRECTIONS:

Wash fruit thoroughly under running water. Cut a zigzag pattern completely around the circumference of the fruit, inserting knife to approximately the center of the fruit. (Refer to diagram below.) For better control, instruct children to hold the knife approximately 1 to 1-1/2" from the tip as they make cuts into the fruit.

Pull fruit apart to expose two fancy "crowns," suitable for a garnish or fancy snack.

Chef Tip: Different fruits can be stacked on top of each other to form a flower.

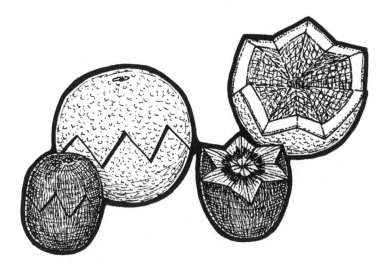

Creative Kebabs

INGREDIENTS/SUPPLIES:

• long wooden skewers or plastic chopsticks (safer for young children), plates

• colorful chunks of fruits or vegetables (see below)

• clean work surface and hands

• Optional: One of the dips on pages 157-158 for vegetable kebabs; Pumpkin pie dip on page 158 for fruit kebabs

Suggested Fruits: Slices/chunks of banana, kiwi, apple, pear, pineapple, melon, orange wedges, star fruit, papaya, strawberries (A spritz of orange or lemon juice will keep fruits such as bananas, apples, and pears from turning brown.)

Suggested Vegetables: Slices/chunks of radishes, cucumber, cherry tomatoes, carrots, broccoli or cauliflower florets, mushrooms, pea pods, summer squash

DIRECTIONS:

Before cutting or slicing, wash all fresh produce thoroughly under running water. Create either fruit or vegetable kebabs by threading chunks or slices onto a wooden skewer. Encourage creative use of color, design and patterning. Discuss how kebabs could be arranged artfully on a platter, placing a bowl of suggested dip in the center.

Chef Tip: Make a bouquet-type display of vegetables by inserting three or four kebabs into a raw potato half. For a fruit bouquet, insert three or four fruit kebabs into a melon half.

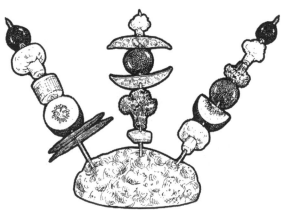

Food Fans

INGREDIENTS/SUPPLIES:

• soft fruit or vegetable such as a fresh peach half, ripe fresh pear half, whole strawberry or a large pickle or cucumber half

• plastic ridged or semi-ridged knives, plates

• clean work surface and hands

DIRECTIONS:

If using fresh produce, wash thoroughly under running water. Place food on work surface so that it is stable (cut "rounded" foods in half to prevent them from rolling). Starting approximately one-half inch from the top, make a cut completely through the fruit or vegetable (see diagram). Make several cuts, parallel to the first one. Press down and "fan out."

Chef Tip: Cucumbers have a great success rate for this garnish. Try making the cuts at an angle across the cucumber for a different effect.

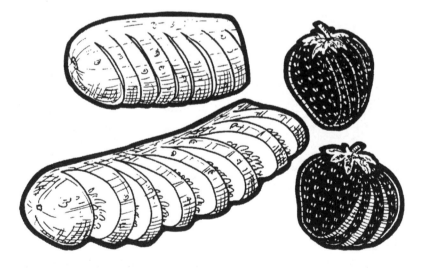

Baby Goose in a Nest Salad

This is a fun way to entice kids to eat salad made from a mixture of fresh greens.

Note: An earlier version of this recipe recommended using sprouts. Because of the possibility of bacterial contamination, government food safety guidelines recommend that children should avoid eating fresh sprouts.

INGREDIENTS/SUPPLIES:

- small or "baby" yellow crooked neck squash, whole cloves, washed and chopped salad greens, orange, low-fat salad dressing

- plastic ridged or semi-ridged knives, plates, forks

- clean work surface and hands

DIRECTIONS:

Wash the orange and salad thoroughly under running water. Cut the orange in half, using the zigzag cut described on page 152. Carefully scoop and/or cut the edible contents out of the orange half, making sure to leave the peel in one piece. Create a "nest" by filling the orange peel with a salad mix such as baby greens or baby spring mix.

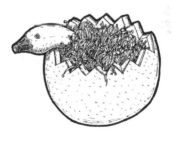

Next, cut the squash off about an inch below the "neck." Insert whole cloves near the stem to make eyes (see diagram). Nestle the goose head and neck into the salad, so it appears the goose is poking out from his nest. If you wish, place two or three squash geese in each nest. Serve with low-fat salad dressing. Be sure to remove the whole cloves before eating the squash.

Note: Eat the orange segments that were scooped out of the peel or chop and mix the orange segments into the salad. The bottom portion of the squash can be sliced and eaten raw, cooked or used in another project.

Chef Tip: Use grapes or grape tomatoes as "eggs" in the nest.

Radish Garnishes

Radishes are frequently used in garnishing because they are inexpensive, colorful and versatile. They are also easy to grow — see Chapter 7, page 109 for instructions. Three examples of radish garnishes are described below.

INGREDIENTS/SUPPLIES:

• radishes, cherry tomatoes, lettuce leaves, whole cloves, uncooked spaghetti, cucumber/carrot peelings

• plastic ridged or semi-ridged knives, plates

• clean work surface and hands

DIRECTIONS:

Before beginning, be sure to thoroughly wash all fresh produce under running water.

Radish Jacks: To make a jack, use two thin slices of radish. Make a single slit to the center point of each slice (the radius). Slip cut ends together to make a jack. To make a display of jacks and a ball, make several radish jacks and use a plump, round radish for the ball.

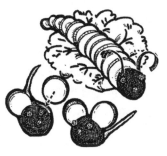

Radish Caterpillar: Using thinly sliced radishes, arrange slices on a lettuce leaf, as shown in diagram. For a head, use a cherry tomato half with cloves for eyes and small pieces of broken spaghetti or thin cucumber or carrot peeling for antennae. Use the same technique to make caterpillars out of sliced carrots or small, sliced cucumbers.

> **Chef Tip:** White icicle radishes work great because they are long. Watch out though — these can taste very hot and spicy!

Radish Mouse: Use a large whole radish with the root (which becomes the tail) still attached. Trim the stem, leaving a small stub for the nose. Use two thin radish slices from another radish for the ears. Make small slits on top of the "head" and insert ears. Use whole cloves for eyes and small pieces of broken spaghetti for whiskers.

Dips

Children are more likely to eat healthful fruits, vegetables and whole grains when they can pair them with a delicious dip. The dips that follow are kid-tested and packed with nutritious ingredients.

Peanut Butter Hummus

INGREDIENTS/SUPPLIES:

- 1 can (15 oz) garbanzo beans, drained and rinsed
  4 tbsp creamy peanut butter, no salt added*
  2 tbsp olive oil
  fresh lemon juice (squeezed from 1 fresh lemon)
  1/3 cup water
  1 tsp garlic powder
  *If a child has a peanut allergy, substitute tahini (sesame paste) for the peanut butter.
- non-breakable mixing bowl, liquid measuring cup, measuring spoons, sharp knife, hand masher
- clean work surface and hands

DIRECTIONS:

Place the garbanzo beans in the bottom of a large non-breakable mixing bowl. Cut a lemon in half and squeeze the lemon juice into a bowl. Begin mashing the beans using the potato masher. If making the recipe with children, allow each child to take a turn mashing the beans. Gradually add the remaining ingredients and continue to mash until the mixture is blended and smooth.

Serve with a colorful assortment of raw vegetables and whole grain crackers. Servings: 10 (approx. 1/4 cup each)
Nutritional information per ¼ cup serving: 118 calories, 4 grams protein, 12 grams carbohydrate, 6 grams fat, 2 grams fiber, 137 milligrams sodium

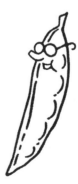

A-B-C Dip (Avocados, Beans, Cilantro)

INGREDIENTS/SUPPLIES:

- 4-5 avocados, peeled and sliced

  1/4 cup finely chopped onion

  1 garlic clove, finely minced

  3 T. fresh lime juice

  1/2 cup chopped fresh tomatoes

  1-15 ounce can black beans, drained and rinsed

  2 tablespoons chopped cilantro

  Salt to taste (optional)

- mixing bowl, sharp knife and cutting board, measuring cup, measuring spoons, hand masher
- clean work surface and hands

DIRECTIONS:

Place avocados, onions, garlic and lime juice into a bowl and mash until slightly lumpy. Stir in tomatoes, beans, and cilantro. If desired, add salt to taste. Serve with a colorful assortment of raw vegetables and whole corn tortilla chips. Servings: 14 (approx. 1/4 cup each)

Nutritional information per ¼ cup serving: 127 calories, 3 grams protein, 11 grams carbo-hydrate, 9 grams fat, 6 grams fiber, 60 milligrams sodium (if made without salt)

Pumpkin Pie Dip

INGREDIENTS/SUPPLIES:

- 6 oz. vanilla Greek yogurt

  2 tbsp. whipped cream cheese

  1/2 cup canned pumpkin

  1 tsp. pumpkin pie spice

  1 Tablespoon honey

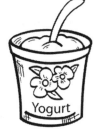

- mixing bowl, measuring cup, measuring spoons, spoon
- clean work surface and hands

DIRECTIONS:

Mix ingredients well and serve with an assortment of colorful fresh cut-up fruit. Servings: 6 (approx. 1/4 cup each)

Nutritional information per ¼ cup serving: 55 calories, 3 grams protein, 8 grams carbohy-drate, 1 gram fat, 1 gram fiber, 34 milligrams sodium

Sandwich Art

The ideas below turn sandwiches into artwork that looks back at you.

Hoagie Faces

INGREDIENTS/SUPPLIES:

• whole grain hoagie buns, sliced low-fat cheeses, lean luncheon or deli meat, shredded carrots or squash, lettuce or baby spinach, olives, cherry tomatoes

• miscellaneous condiments (mustard, reduced-fat mayonnaise, low-fat Italian dressing, etc.)

• toothpicks or broken spaghetti pieces, plates

• clean work surface and hands

DIRECTIONS:

Make hoagie sandwich, using desired ingredients. On one end of the sandwich, use toothpicks or broken spaghetti pieces to position olives for eyeballs, and a cherry tomato for the nose. Arrange shredded carrots or squash on top for hair (see diagram). If desired, make a tongue by sticking a small piece of lunch meat out of the "mouth."

Note: Be sure to remove all toothpicks or spaghetti pieces before eating.

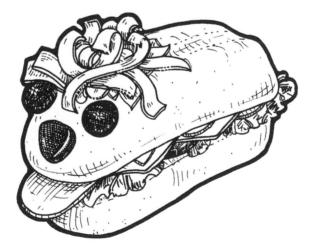

Smiling Burritos

INGREDIENTS/SUPPLIES:

• whole grain flour or corn tortilla, refried beans, grated part-skim mozzarella cheese, black olives, cherry tomato, kidney or black beans, orange wedges

• salsa (optional)

• microwave-safe plates, spoons

• clean work surface and hands

DIRECTIONS:

Spread refried beans on tortilla. Use remaining ingredients to make a smiling face: cheese for hair, olives for eyes, a cherry tomato nose and bean smile. Microwave on high for 30 seconds - 1 minute. Place orange wedges beside the burrito for ears. If desired, serve with salsa.

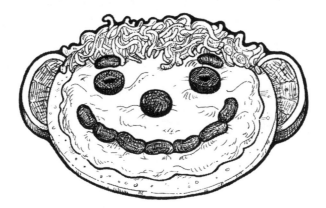

Tuna Mandarin Roll-Ups

Spice up ordinary tuna salad with curry powder and sweet, colorful Mandarin oranges.

INGREDIENTS/SUPPLIES:

- 1 can (12 ounces) tuna in water, drained
  ¼ cup reduced-fat mayonnaise
  ¼ teaspoon curry powder
  1 can (11 ounces) Mandarin orange segments, drained
  1/3 cup finely chopped celery
  4 medium whole grain tortillas or flatbread
  2 cups lettuce or baby spinach leaves

- measuring cups and spoons, fork, spoon, mixing bowl, plates

- clean work surface and hands

DIRECTIONS:

In medium bowl, use fork to combine tuna, mayonnaise and curry powder. Mix well. Stir in oranges and celery. Spread ½ cup tuna mixture onto each tortilla or flatbread to within 1 inch of edge; top with ½ cup lettuce or baby spinach leaves. Roll up; serve immediately.

Adapted with permission from the Canned Food Alliance, located at www.mealtime.org.

Servings: 4

Nutritional information per serving: 250 calories, 25 grams protein, 28 grams carbohydrate, 3.5 grams fat, 3 grams fiber, 620 milligrams sodium

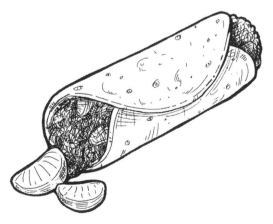

Pizza Faces

INGREDIENTS/SUPPLIES:

- whole grain English muffins or bagel halves (split open), prepared pizza or spaghetti sauce, grated part-skim mozzarella cheese, vegetables such as sliced olives, sliced mushrooms, red pepper rings, chopped onions and broccoli florets

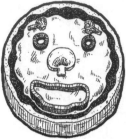

- spoons, plates

- baking tray and oven or toaster oven

- clean work surface and hands

DIRECTIONS:

Spread an English muffin half with pizza sauce and top with mozzarella cheese. Using the vegetables, create a "face" design. Broil 3-4 minutes or until cheese is golden and bubbly.

Chef Tip: Adapt this activity for special holidays. Make Jack-O'-Lantern, Santa, Cupid or Leprechaun pizza faces.

Fresh Faces

INGREDIENTS/SUPPLIES:

- whole grain toaster waffles or English muffins (split open), nut butter or reduced fat cream cheese, pineapple tidbits, sunflower seeds, raisins, berries and banana slices

- plastic knives, plates

- clean work surface and hands

DIRECTIONS:

Spread toasted waffle or muffin half with peanut butter or cream cheese. Using remaining ingredients, make a face, pattern or other art design.

Bread Dough Art

Using bread dough, children can create virtually any shape, letter, animal or design that they wish. It's as versatile as clay and a lot more delicious.

INGREDIENTS/SUPPLIES:

• frozen whole grain bread dough, unbaked roll or bread dough from the school cafeteria or bread dough made from scratch

• plates, baking tray, parchment paper and oven

• clean work surface and hands

DIRECTIONS:

If dough is frozen, thaw beforehand. On a floured surface, divide dough into individual portions. Pass out to children, instructing them to roll, knead and shape dough into desired shapes. Place on cookie sheet lined with parchment baking paper, labeling each child's creation. Preheat oven to 375°F. Let rise, uncovered, for 15–20 minutes in a warm, draft-free place. Bake bread on center shelf of oven for 15–20 minutes (until golden brown). Cooking time will vary depending on shape and thickness of art.

Optional: Discuss the scientific principles involved in bread baking, including how yeast causes bread to rise and predictions about how the art will change during the baking process.

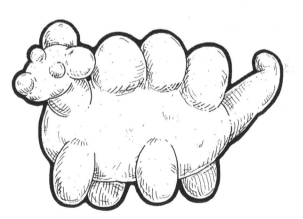

Very Berry Frozen Pops

These colorful, tasty pops can be garnished with fresh berries or a fanned-out strawberry from page 154.

INGREDIENTS/SUPPLIES:

• 1 cup flavored low-fat yogurt (try blueberry, vanilla, or lemon)

• 1 cup fresh or thawed frozen berries (blueberries, strawberries, raspberries, or a mixture of all three)

• 4 3-ounce paper cups

• 4 plastic spoons

• Measuring cup, mixing bowl, fork or masher

• clean work surface and hands

DIRECTIONS:

In medium bowl, mash berries with a fork or masher until they are a smooth consistency. Add the yogurt and mix well. Divide the mixture evenly between the four paper cups. Stick a plastic spoon in the middle. Freeze for two hours or until the pops are solid. Peel off the paper cup and enjoy!

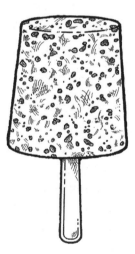

Makes 4 frozen pops.

Nutritional information per serving: 56 calories, 3 grams protein, 11 grams carbohydrate, 0 grams fat, 2 grams fiber, 40 milligrams sodium

Yummy Pumpkin Softies

These delicious soft cookies contain nutritious ingredients. Kids can use dried fruit and nuts to create their own designer cookies.

INGREDIENTS/SUPPLIES:

- 1 ½ cups firmly packed brown sugar
  ½ cup trans-fat free margarine or butter
  1 can (15 ounces) pumpkin
  2 eggs
  2 ½ cups whole wheat pastry flour
  1 teaspoon baking powder
  ½ teaspoon baking soda
  1 teaspoon ground cinnamon
  ½ teaspoon salt
  ⅛ teaspoon ground nutmeg
  Nonstick spray

- Toppings: raisins, dried cranberries, sliced or slivered almonds, walnuts, chopped dried prunes or apricots

- spoon, 2 mixing bowls, baking sheet, measuring cups and spoons

- clean work surface and hands

DIRECTIONS:

Preheat oven to 350°F. In mixing bowl, beat together sugar and trans-fat free margarine until creamy. Add pumpkin and eggs; beat well. In medium bowl, combine flour, baking powder, baking soda, cinnamon, salt and nutmeg; add to pumpkin mixture, mixing until dry ingredients are moistened. Spray a baking sheet with nonstick spray. Drop dough by rounded measuring tablespoonfuls onto pan. Smooth tops of dough with back of spoon and decorate with dried fruits and nuts to make flowers, faces or other fun patterns. Bake 15 to 18 minutes or until bottoms are golden brown. Remove to wire racks; cool completely. Makes about 3-1/2 dozen.

Adapted with permission from the Canned Food Alliance, located at www.mealtime.org.
Nutritional information per cookie: 80 calories, 1 gram protein, 14 grams carbohydrate, 2.5 grams fat, 1 gram fiber, 60 milligrams sodium

Cookie Cutter Fun

Cookie cutters can be used with food in many imaginative ways. Designs are especially fun when they complement thematic units or parties.

DIRECTIONS:

Fun-Shaped Sandwiches: Cut sandwiches with soft fillings such as cheese, nut butters, egg or tuna salad into fun shapes. Don't waste the outside edges — they can be cut into small finger sandwiches.

Breakfast Art: Use cookie cutters to make fun-shaped pancakes, waffles or French toast. To make a fun "egg in the toast," cut a shape out of the center of a slice of bread, lightly butter both sides and place in a non-stick pan. Crack an egg into the center of the bread. Once the egg sets, carefully flip over and continue cooking until the egg is thoroughly cooked.

Cheese Shapes: Cut cheese slices into various shapes and arrange on a platter with crackers. Or, melt cheese shapes onto dark bread or toast to make unique open-faced toasted cheese sandwiches.

Contrasting Cutouts: Using either light and dark breads (light rye and pumpernickel work well) or a variety of ½" melon slices (e.g. watermelon, cantaloupe and honeydew), create contrasting designs with cookie cutters. Carefully cut identical sections out of slices of bread or melon. Reverse the cutouts to create colorful contrasts (see diagram).

Indentations: On the top of sandwiches, melon slices, thick Greek yogurt or even cooked brown rice, press cookie cutter lightly until an indentation is visible.

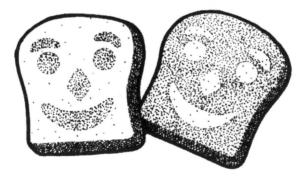

Expanding on Edible Art

The following ideas can be assigned as homework or included as suggestions in a parent newsletter.

▲ At home, encourage children to garnish a serving platter, salad bowl or individual plates as a way to make family dinners extra special.

▲ Older children may want to host or cater an event for their friends. Birthday or holiday parties, post-game get-togethers or even "break the boredom" events are all chances for kids to impress their friends with their savvy food skills.

▲ Snacktime becomes learning and fun time when students prepare food in fancy ways. Children may actually eat a more varied diet when they have a hand in making fun food creations.

▣ At school, students can make fancy garnishes for the cafeteria serving line or self-service variety bars.

▲ Invite a local chef to come to the classroom and teach students additional garnishes and cooking skills, expose children to careers in the culinary field and reinforce nutrition concepts. A resource for finding local chefs to partner with is the *Chefs Move to Schools* initiative. For more information, visit www.chefsmovetoschools.org.

▲ Encourage children to expand their culinary skills by checking out one of the kids' cookbooks listed in Appendix B.

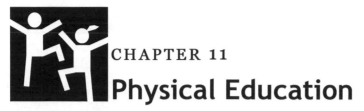

CHAPTER 11
Physical Education

If I were a car, I wouldn't get far
Without some gas, so please pass
Some human fuel (known as food),
To fill my tank and improve my mood!
       —CLE

Food is only one part of the fitness equation. The optimal growth and development of young bodies requires movement, play, exercise and rest. A successful school-based physical fitness program emphasizes fun, fitness and the attainment of life skills.

Children who are active feel better, have more energy and even learn more easily than their sedentary peers. A strong physical education program, along with a solid nutrition program, boosts the entire school learning environment. Children in good physical condition bring more focus, stamina and creativity to the classroom.

Nutrition principles are naturally integrated into the study and practice of physical education. Presented here are activities which reinforce the role diet and exercise play in heart health, the importance of goal setting when targeting health behaviors, the best foods to eat for sports and play, active games that reinforce nutrition and fitness concepts and

Fit Kids are Smarter Kids

There is a distinct relationship between academic achievement and physical fitness, according to a report from the Centers for Disease Control and Prevention (CDC). The key findings:

♦ There is substantial evidence that physical activity can help improve academic achievement (including grades and standardized test scores).

♦ Physical activity can have an impact on cognitive skills, attitudes and academic behavior, all of which are important components of improved academic performance. These include enhanced concentration and attention as well as improved classroom behavior.

♦ The report recommends that schools employ a number of strategies to increase children's physical activity including school-based physical education, recess, classroom-based physical activity and extracurricular physical activities.

Centers for Disease Control and Prevention, U.S. Department of Health and Human Services. (2010). The association between school based physical activity, including physical education, and academic performance.

advice from one teacher who integrates walking into all aspects of her curriculum.

🏃 Taking Care of the Hard Working Heart

The strongest muscle in the body, the heart pumps an average of 2,000 gallons of blood each day. Because it is a muscle, the heart becomes stronger and more efficient when it is exercised regularly.

> Every day, children should engage in at least one hour of moderate to vigorous physical activity such as P.E., organized sports or active play.

Diet also plays a vital role in keeping the heart healthy. While nutrition scientists continue to search for definitive answers about diet and heart health, they do know that a high intake of saturated fat, trans fat, and to a lesser degree, dietary cholesterol, places many people at increased risk for heart disease. When the concentration of cholesterol in the blood runs consistently high, fatty deposits eventually build up in the **coronary arteries**, the blood vessels that supply the heart with oxygen and nutrients. When a coronary artery becomes completely blocked with fat, the blood supply to that section of the heart muscle is shut off, resulting in the life-threatening event known as a heart attack.

Limiting fat is only one piece of a heart smart lifestyle, though. Eating an overall well-balanced diet — rich in high-fiber grains, beans, fruits and vegetables — lowers the risk of heart disease. Also vital to heart health are lifetime habits that include regular exercise, relaxation, a tobacco-free lifestyle and the control of blood pressure.

THE HEART

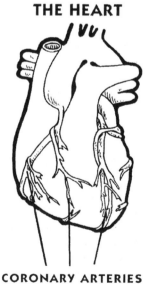

CORONARY ARTERIES

While it is the rare child who will experience coronary heart disease in youth, autopsy and imaging studies show that the development of fatty arteries begins in childhood. Clearly, the best "cure" for heart disease involves adopting healthful habits starting at an early age.

Table 11-1

Fat Facts

- Fat is essential to health, development and growth.

- In the body, fat serves as a shock absorber that protects internal organs, aids in temperature regulation, provides insulation, serves as an energy reservoir and comprises an important part of the cell membrane.

- In the diet, fat provides the essential fatty acids which are alpha-linolenic acid (ALA) and linoleic acid. Dietary fat also aids in the transport and absorption of the fat-soluble vitamins (A, D, E and K).

- Fat plays an important role in promoting growth and development in infants. Breast milk derives more than half of its calories from fat and is high in cholesterol as well.

- Fat tastes good and provides a feeling of satisfaction. Since fat is digested more slowly than carbohydrate or protein, it delays feelings of hunger between meals.

- Fat contains nine calories per gram, while the other energy nutrients — carbohydrate and protein — each contain four calories per gram.

- A high level of cholesterol in the blood is a major risk factor for coronary artery disease. Both trans fat and saturated fat have been linked to high blood cholesterol levels. Dietary cholesterol has only a moderate effect on blood cholesterol levels in some people.

- The 2010 Dietary Guidelines for Americans recommend that children ages 4 to 18 eat 25-35 percent of their total calories from fat. The guidelines also recommend that most Americans should avoid trans fat, consume 10 percent or fewer of their calories from saturated fat and limit cholesterol to no more than 300 milligrams each day.

TYPES OF FAT:

- **Saturated fats** are solid at room temperature and include the fats found in most animal products (meat, dairy products and eggs) and certain vegetable oils (e.g. coconut oil, palm kernel oil, cocoa butter).

- **Trans fats** are oils that have been chemically altered through a process called hydrogenation to make them more saturated. See page 88 for more about trans fat.

- **Monounsaturated fats,** found in foods such as olive oil, peanut oil, canola oil, olives, peanuts, nuts and avocados, tend to lower total blood cholesterol and Low Density Lipoproteins (LDL) while maintaining the levels of "good" cholesterol know as High Density Lipoproteins (HDL). HDLs carry cholesterol from the coronary arteries back to the liver where it is broken down. (Regular aerobic exercise is the best way to increase HDL levels.)

- **Polyunsaturated fats** are also known to lower cholesterol and include oils such as corn, safflower, soybean and sunflower seed. **Omega-3** fatty acids are a unique type of polyunsaturated fat that show promise in promoting heart health. Flaxseed oil, walnuts and fatty fish (particularly the cold water varieties such as mackerel, salmon, sardines and tuna) are rich in omega-3 fatty acids.

- **Cholesterol** is a waxy fatlike substance produced by the body and consumed in the diet. Blood cholesterol levels vary between individuals and are influenced by both genetics and diet. Dietary cholesterol is found only in animal foods. Full-fat dairy products, egg yolks, animal fat and liver are the most common sources of dietary cholesterol.

HEART RATE

Teach children to monitor their heart or pulse rates using their index and middle fingers on either the wrist or neck (carotid pulse). An easy way to find the carotid pulse is to place the thumb of the right hand on the chin and then search with the first two fingers until the pulse feels strong and steady. Time the pulse for six seconds, instructing children when to start and stop counting. Multiply the number times 10 for the beats-per-minute pulse rate.

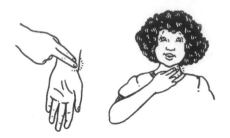

ACTIVITIES

▲ Contrast resting heart rate with active heart rate. (The resting heart rate for an average child is around 80 beats per minute.) Have children take their pulse at rest and record. Next, have them jump rope or run in place for 1-2 minutes, checking pulse immediately after they finish. What happens to the pulse rate?

▲ Ask students to keep a pulse rate chart, noting how their heart rate responds to different situations, such as waking up, after eating, when scared or nervous, during active play or before bed.

> **Laqueesha's Pulse Rate**
>
> When I wake up __73__
> At a scary movie __94__
> After riding my bike __120__
> Doing Homework __82__

▲ Assign students math problems which use their pulse data. For instance, using resting pulse rate, calculate how many times the heart beats each day, week, month, etc. How many extra beats does 30 minutes of exercise or active play add to the total each day? Does the resting pulse rate vary between children in the class? Are there differences between girls and boys? Plot the results in a table or show graphically.

▲ Pose the following "challenge question" to students: Will a heart made strong through regular exercise beat faster or slower when at rest? (ANSWER: The resting heart rate is slower because a strong heart can pump more blood with fewer beats. Many endurance athletes have resting pulse rates as low as 40 beats per minute.)

▲ Target heart rate is the pulse rate to strive for during aerobic activities. An aerobic activity uses large muscle groups and includes activities such as running, jumping rope, swimming, biking and soccer. To build cardiorespiratory endurance, it is recommended that children exercise at their target heart rates (shown in Table 11-2) a minimum of 20 continuous minutes on most days of the week.

Cardiorespiratory endurance is the ability of the heart, lungs and blood vessels to deliver oxygen to hard working muscles.

Table 11-2

Target Heart Rate	
Resting Rate	**Target Rate**
below 60	150
60-64	151
65-69	152
70-74	153
75-79	155
80-84	159
85-89	161
90 & above	163

Source: Hopper, C., Fisher, B., & Munoz, K. (2008). *Physical activity and nutrition for health*. Champaign, IL: Human Kinetics.

EATING FOR A HEALTHY HEART

Discuss how *MyPlate* can be a helpful tool in planning a heart-healthy diet which includes plenty of colorful fruits and vegetables, whole grains, low-fat dairy and lean protein foods such as seafood and beans. Ask children to list choices from each food group that contribute to heart health. Point out how some choices in the dairy and protein group vary greatly in their saturated fat content. For instance, contrast the saturated fat content of skinless baked chicken and fried chicken, whole and 1% milk, ground beef and dried beans or fat-free yogurt and cheese.

ACTIVITIES

▲ Using the blank *MyPlate* on page 52, have students design their personal version of a heart-healthy *MyPlate*.

You Will Need:
♦ *Nutrition Facts* label information from a variety of foods

▲ Ask students why they think the *Nutrition Facts* food label contains information on saturated fat and trans fat. (ANSWER: Saturated and trans fat have the most direct link to high blood cholesterol levels.) Visit a grocery store or bring in a variety of food labels and compare saturated and trans fat contents. Examples include butter and margarine, different types of milk, a variety of cheeses, labels from meat products and snack items such as cookies and crackers.

▲ **How Fat Clogs Arteries:** Utilize the classroom water table or rubber basins to emulate the process of how fat affects arteries. You will need clear plastic tubing, solid vegetable shortening, cotton swabs and red food coloring. Fill the water table or basin with water; add red food coloring. Explain

You Will Need:
♦ Clear, flexible tubing
♦ Solid vegetable shortening
♦ Cotton swabs
♦ Red food coloring
♦ Water table or rubber basin

to the students that the water represents blood, the tubes are arteries and the shortening is fat that deposits in the arteries. Children can play and experiment, noting how a dab of fat in the tubing impairs "blood flow" and what happens when the tubing is totally blocked with fat. (Reassure children that the process of fat accumulation in the arteries takes many years and is not the result of an occasional fatty meal.)

Goal Setting

When making any kind of habit change, it's important to set a goal and keep track of progress. This is especially true for health behaviors, since they involve changing daily habits. Children, especially those younger than age 12, have a definite advantage since their lifetime habits are still under construction.

ACTIVITY

▲ Encourage children to set weekly health, nutrition or fitness goals. It is important to record progress toward the goal, which can be as simple as a checkmark on a chart, a daily bar to color on a graph or a simple entry in a health journal. Consider individual as well as classroom goals.

Examples of individual goals might be to participate in active play after school at least 20 minutes, four days a week or choose a heart-healthy after school snack each day. Classroom goals might consist of five minutes of daily relaxation, a minimum of two 20 minute classroom walks each week or a commitment to eat breakfast every day.

Goals should be simple, achievable and easy to measure. It is also important to reward achieved goals. Non-food rewards are best and can range from classroom privileges, extra recess time, stickers, bookmarks and pencils to business-donated items such as movie passes, water bottles or gift certificates.

> **Check this out:**
> *Nutrition Fun with Brocc & Roll* by Connie Liakos Evers is the companion activity guide to this book. The *Setting Goals and Making Choices* chapter includes activity sheets and a calendar which features the S.N.A.C.K. goal setting system (Small, Needed, Achievable, Counting, Know-How).

Eating for Exercise

THE BEST FUEL

Active kids do best when they fuel their bodies with nutrient-rich carbohydrates. During exercise, carbohydrate fuels the hard-working muscles via the breakdown of **glycogen**, which is the storage form of carbohydrate that releases glucose during muscle work. The body also relies on a steady stream of blood glucose to fuel all body systems, even the brain.

The best way to replenish the body's carbohydrate stores is to eat a diet rich in whole grains, beans, fruits and vegetables. The more active the child, the more carbohydrate is needed for refueling. Fatigue, "burn out" and lack of stamina can all be signs that body carbohydrate stores are low. It's important to note that while sugars are also a type of carbohydrate (known as simple carbohydrates), sugary foods provide a quick burst of energy but little in the way of nutrition. Complex carbohydrates provide a more sustained source of energy.

Active kids also need a continuous supply of fuel throughout the day. Encourage students to begin every day with breakfast, fuel up with a healthy lunch at school and make healthy snack choices.

ACTIVITY

Create analogies between the active body and an automobile. Have the children expand and explain the similarities, using the following examples: Gasoline is to a car like (food) is to a body; a body that runs out of carbohydrate is like a car that runs out of (gasoline); filling a car with high-octane fuel is like feeding the athlete with a high-(carbohydrate) diet; an engine is fueled by gasoline in the same way the working (muscles) are fueled by carbohydrates.

Encourage children to write and illustrate stories that show the analogy between fueling a car and feeding a body.

THE MOST IMPORTANT NUTRIENT

Water is the nutrient of most immediate concern to the young athlete. During training or competition, thirst is not a good indicator of fluid needs. Not only will dehydration impair a child's performance, it also poses a severe, immediate health risk. Frequent water breaks, especially in warm weather, are a necessity. Each pound of water lost through sweat should be replaced with 16 ounces (2 cups) of fluid.

Children should be encouraged to drink before, during and after practice and events. Plain water is the best choice, since it is cheap and readily available. Sugary beverages and juice are not good choices because they slow the absorption of water from the stomach into the body. A sports drink is recommended only when exercising in the heat or participating in activities that last longer than 90 minutes.

ACTIVITIES

As homework, ask children to weigh themselves before and after active play, a sporting event or other physical activity. Have each child calculate how much weight was lost. (**Note:** Due to sensitivity around weight issues, the students should not report actual weight, just the difference in weight before and after the activity). Explain that the weight change was due to water loss from perspiration. Ask children to calculate how much fluid they should drink to replace the loss. For more accurate results, instruct children to use the restroom before weighing and monitor fluids consumed during the activity.

▲ Have students keep a record of fluid intake throughout the day. Include water, juice, milk and other beverages as well as less obvious sources such as frozen treats, soup and other liquid foods.

Ask students if they know how to tell whether they are drinking enough fluids. Explain that by the time we experience thirst, the body may already be mildly dehydrated. The best way to check hydration is to make sure urine is clear to light yellow.

During the busy school day, children often forget to drink fluids. Remind students to drink water at recess, before or after breaks and at lunchtime.

PRE-EVENT EATING

What and when a young athlete eats can influence the outcome of practice or the big game. The hard-working muscles should be well fueled for activity. This is accomplished with a meal that is eaten two to three hours prior to the start of an event. On practice days, a snack or light meal can be eaten up to one hour before.

It is best to have the stomach nearly empty during sports and vigorous physical activity. Normally, blood is diverted to the vessels surrounding the digestive tract right after eating. Likewise, physical activity requires a lion's share of the blood to supply exercising muscles with fuel and oxygen. Exercising with a full stomach stages a competition between the muscles and digestive tract, resulting in poor physical performance as well as an upset stomach.

Foods high in complex carbohydrates, moderate in protein and low in fat and sugar are ideal for pre-exercise meals. The energy in sugar is short-lived while greasy foods hang in the stomach for hours (see Chapter 7, page 103, for an explanation of fat digestion). Fluids should also be emphasized prior to physical activity.

Good nutrition is also important after the game. This is the time to replenish the body's stores of carbohydrate and other key nutrients with a healthful, balanced meal that includes 4-5 food groups.

ACTIVITIES

You Will Need:

♦ *Nutrition Facts* label information for foods used in the digestion race activity

▲ Using the board or classroom projector, stage a "digestion race," where students determine which foods they think will take longer to leave their stomachs. Pair foods with identical serving sizes, but varying amounts of fat. Examples include baked pita chips versus potato chips, a whole wheat mini-bagel versus a doughnut, high-fat versus low-fat crackers or ice cream versus fat-free yogurt.

Ask students to explain the differences between the two foods, noting which takes longer to digest and why. Share *Nutrition Facts* label information from the products with students, asking them to note the fat content of the two foods. Discuss which food is better to eat before exercise.

▲ Assign students the task of planning a pre-event meal. Meals should be high in complex carbohydrate, moderate in protein, low in fat, low in added sugar and paired with a beverage. Students can get ideas from the sample meals listed in Table 11-3.

Table 11-3

Pre-Exercise Meal Ideas

The pre-event meals below can be eaten 1 hour before a light practice or recreational activity and 2-3 hours before vigorous activity or competitive sporting events. Add a glass of low-fat milk or water to complete the meal.

- Turkey sandwich on whole grain bread with lettuce, tomato slices, Swiss cheese, a dab of light mayonnaise or mustard; apple slices

- Baked potato topped with black beans, salsa and a sprinkle of grated cheddar cheese; kiwi slices

- Grilled salmon, brown rice and small green salad with low-fat dressing

- Whole grain Pita bread stuffed with tuna, baby greens, cucumber slices and a dab of light mayonnaise; grapes

- Whole grain English muffin split and topped with pizza sauce, pepper rings, mushroom slices, olives and part-skim mozzarella (broil or microwave to melt cheese); melon slices

- Peanut butter & fruit sandwich on whole-wheat bread (try sliced banana, sliced fresh peach or raisins)

- Corn tortilla topped with hot refried beans, a sprinkle of cheese, shredded lettuce, diced tomato and avocado chunks

- Whole grain pasta with marinara sauce, a sprinkle of Parmesan cheese and baby carrots

- Bowl of lean beef vegetable soup and whole grain crackers

Suggest that students interview a local high school, college or professional athlete about his or her diet. The student should find out what the athlete typically eats in a day, favorite foods, meals eaten before competition, foods the athlete avoids and any special food or nutrition habits that help the athlete to perform better. Ask the student to write a report and/or present the information to the class. (But keep in mind that sometimes even the best athletes don't always practice good nutrition.)

Food Games

Active games that promote nutrition concepts can be creative, fun and educational. The following games reinforce the principles of *MyPlate* as students engage in active play. Encourage children to develop their own active games that center on a food or nutrition theme.

ACTIVITIES

▲ **Let's Make a Meal Relay:** Reproduce the food group cards on page 181, cut them out and place them in a hat. Adjust the number of cards according to group size. The game is based on multiples of 5 so you may need to have some students take turns sitting out and serving as monitors.

Have each student draw a card from the hat while not looking. The monitors can make sure that no one in the group peeks at the cards before the game begins. The objective is for students to form a relay team made up of five members, with each student on the team representing a different food group.

Explain that when you blow your whistle (or yell "Go"), students are to mingle, share with classmates which food group they represent and organize into "complete meal" teams made of all five food groups. (Warning: This is a noisy game!) Once a team is assembled, each team member will run an assigned length, relay style. The first team to finish is the winner. Repeat the game until everyone has a chance to play.

> **Going further:** Make the game more challenging by having the finishing team members hold up their card and give an example of a food in their food group.

▲ **Build a MyPlate Scramble:** Similar to the meal relay, students will again draw food group slips out of a hat. The objective is for the students to

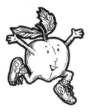 scramble and organize themselves into a circle that matches the formation of the *MyPlate* food guide. Refer to page 53 for placement of the food groups in *MyPlate*. Use a stopwatch to time students, noting their improvement with subsequent efforts.

Food Group Cards

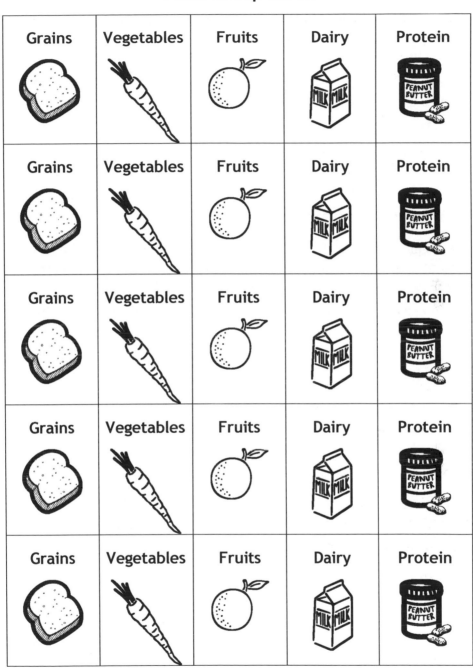

Grains	Vegetables	Fruits	Dairy	Protein
Grains	Vegetables	Fruits	Dairy	Protein
Grains	Vegetables	Fruits	Dairy	Protein
Grains	Vegetables	Fruits	Dairy	Protein
Grains	Vegetables	Fruits	Dairy	Protein

Reproduce, cut apart and use in food group games.

▲ **Jump Rope Jingles:** Ask students to invent jingles with a nutrition twist. For example, "Eating *MyPlate* at my dinner, name each group and be the winner," followed by the child calling out a different food group for each jump (e.g., rice/jump, carrots/jump, peach/jump, chicken/jump, milk/jump). The goal is to name a food from a different food group with every jump. (It's harder than it first appears.)

Encourage students to put a new twist on old favorites. For example, "Cinderella dressed in teal; Went inside to eat her meal; How many _____ (insert food group name here) did she eat?" Call out the names of foods that are in the selected food group with a different food corresponding to each jump.

▲**Veggie, Veggie, Fruit (or Fruit, Fruit, Veggie):** Targeted to younger children, this is a variation of the traditional Duck, Duck, Goose game. The children will sit in a circle and one child will be the leader. Walking around the circle, the leader will tap each child as a veggie or a fruit. When the leader taps a child as a fruit, this child will get up and chase the leader around the circle. If the child tags the leader before he or she gets to the original spot, the leader will continue the game. Otherwise, the tagged child will become the new leader.

To make the game more educational and challenging, have the leader name specific vegetables and fruits. For instance, the leader will tap the children with vegetable names such as carrot, broccoli, peas and lettuce. The leader will tap a child with "fruit" by naming a specific fruit such as apple, peach, banana or grapes.

The Walking Classroom

According to Carolyn Johnson, a Portland, Oregon, elementary teacher, "just about anything you teach in the classroom can be done on a walk."

Carolyn, a serious walker herself, takes her classroom beyond four walls by integrating walking into all areas of her curriculum. She divides walking into three categories: fitness walking, "taking a break" walking and walking field trips and games.

FITNESS WALKING

When Carolyn takes her class on a fitness walk, she emphasizes a pace that is consistent, steady and relatively uninterrupted. She works on warming up, cooling down, stretching, appropriate pacing and good posture with her students. During fitness walks, she exposes her class to different walking paces and varying terrain.

On soggy Oregon days that are too wet for an outside walk, Carolyn sets up a classroom fitness circuit.

TAKE A BREAK

Carolyn takes her class on short walks as a type of mental break. "Studies show that short walks can give us an energy boost and help to improve our mood," states Johnson. She gives her class walking breaks before an assembly when quiet sitting will be expected, when they need a "breather" and when they have been working hard and need a change of pace. She also walks with her class the first few minutes of each recess.

DISCOVERY WALKS

Carolyn incorporates academics into walking by taking discovery field trips around the school neighborhood. Her students become meteorologists by observing, graphing and measuring weather; monitoring the evaporation rates of puddles and creating big books based on their findings. They watch trees change throughout the seasons; note different colors, shapes and sounds and observe different forms of transportation. After a visit to a farm, her class walks to a neighborhood grocery store to see where the harvested food goes (and later develop a classroom grocery store based on their newfound knowledge).

Carolyn naturally incorporates her teaching of nutrition and healthful lifestyle habits into her classroom walks. "Perhaps the greatest reward from our daily walks is the growth of each child's self-esteem. Everyone is successful at walking and everyone has fun."

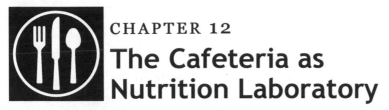

CHAPTER 12
The Cafeteria as Nutrition Laboratory

"I'm looking forward to coming and seeing the central kitchen. I like the food that your factory cooks." — *Jonathan*

As the nutrition lesson I was presenting came to a close, one of the first graders invited me to stay and eat lunch with her. Soon, several more children chimed in, pleading for me to be their guest in the school cafeteria. Curious to experience school lunch from a new perspective, I agreed.

As we crowded together to eat, I felt surrounded by adults giving directions over a microphone, pacing up and down the aisles and hurrying each table off to play. My "classmates" warned me not to talk too much or too loudly. Before I had eaten half my meal, the cafeteria monitor excused our entire table! An eye-opening experience, lunch that day was a powerful reminder of how adult order and rules can sometimes bypass the needs of children.

Lunch is much more than a routine break in the middle of the school day. The cafeteria can be an integral part of the education of students — offering children firsthand experience with nutritious food choices, a chance to socialize with friends and a pleasant atmosphere to recharge body and mind.

This visionary cafeteria is possible but requires time, effort and education to succeed. Training for nutrition staff, a commitment from school faculty and administration and support from parents and the community all contribute to a successful school meal program.

Presented here are ideas on how every school cafeteria can become a center for nutrition education. Of primary importance is a menu that features choices consistent with the 2010 Dietary Guidelines for Americans. Students entering the cafeteria can then easily recognize *MyPlate* in action. This chapter also provides suggestions on how to enhance mealtime atmosphere and successfully market the school meal program.

For those worried about skin-tight budgets, the ideas outlined in this chapter make good business sense, too. A solid nutrition program — marketed right — increases participation and boosts image. A number of school cafeterias throughout the country have successfully advanced their programs by making health-minded changes.

School Meals:
An Important Part of a Healthy School Environment

LOCAL SCHOOL WELLNESS POLICIES

Beginning with school year 2006-2007, all local education agencies (LEA) participating in the National School Lunch Program (NSLP) were required by law to establish a local school wellness policy. The policies had to include goals for nutrition education, physical activity and other school-based activities that promote student wellness, as well as nutrition guidelines to promote student health and reduce childhood obesity. Unfortunately, preliminary studies have shown that the policies have been inconsistent in quality and in many cases, have not been properly implemented or evaluated.

The Healthy, Hunger-Free Kids Act of 2010, which reauthorized federal child nutrition programs, also aims to strengthen local school wellness policies. The new act requires ongoing implementation and assessment of policies, factors that were lacking in the initial legislation. Another goal is to include more members from the community in wellness policy development. LEAs will be required to allow physical education teachers and school health professionals as well as parents, students, school nutrition directors, the school board, school administrators, and the public to participate in the process.

SCHOOL MEALS

School meals have shown improvement in recent years, according to the School Nutrition Dietary Assessment-III (SNDA-III). For instance, in school year 2004-2005, school lunches in most schools met USDA goals for target nutrients and were lower in saturated fat than meals offered and served in school year 1998-1999. The SNDA-III also found that students who ate school lunch consumed more nutrients than students who did not participate in the NSLP.

A 2012 report from the Robert Wood Johnson Foundation found that elementary schools have made whole grain products and low-fat milks more available during lunch, but there has been no increase in the availability of salads or fresh fruits. The report also noted that most elementary schools continued to regularly offer high fat foods such as pizza and fried potato products.

As the new nutrition standards outlined in the Healthy, Hunger-Free Kids Act are fully implemented, students should see continued improvement in the nutritional quality of their school meals. The new nutrition standards:

- ◆ Ensure that students are offered both fruits and vegetables every day of the week

- ◆ Substantially increase offerings of whole grain-rich foods

- ◆ Allow only fat-free or low-fat milk varieties

- ◆ Limit calories based on the age of children being served to ensure proper portion size

- ◆ Increase the focus on reducing the amounts of saturated fat, trans fats and sodium.

COMPETITIVE FOODS

While the nutritional quality of school meals has shown improvement in recent years, the overall school environment for healthy eating lags behind. The reason is primarily due to the continued availability of "competitive foods," (i.e., foods offered at schools that are not part of the USDA school meal programs). Examples include food items sold from vending machines, student stores, after-school fundraisers and a la carte sales in the cafeteria. While it is possible to serve healthful choices from these venues, the reality is that most of the competitive foods marketed to children fall into the "empty calorie" category. A recent study reported that nearly half of elementary students in the U.S. could buy unhealthy snacks such as cookies, cakes and baked goods at school during the 2009–10 school year.

A ground-breaking provision in the Healthy, Hunger-Free Kids Act gives USDA the authority to set nutritional standards for all foods regularly sold in schools during the school day, including vending machines, the "a la carte" lunch lines, and school stores. This is an important step forward and hopefully, will facilitate an eating environment where children are not enticed to choose empty calorie foods and beverages over healthy meals and snacks.

WHAT SCHOOLS CAN DO

It is ultimately up to each individual school to make changes that support a healthy school environment. For starters, score your nutrition program using the self-assessment checklist in Table 12-1. This "checklist for success" is a quick, helpful tool to evaluate your nutrition program and set goals for improvement.

For a more comprehensive assessment of your school's overall health environment, a useful tool is *The School Health Index (SHI): Self-Assessment & Planning Guide* from the Centers for Disease Control and Prevention, available at www.cdc.gov/healthyyouth/shi/index.htm. Another recommended assessment tool is the *Healthy Schools Program Inventory* available from the Alliance for a Healthier Generation, which is located at schools.healthiergeneration.org.

Initiatives and organizations that focus on school meals as an important component of a healthy school environment are highlighted in Table 12-2. Appendix B also includes a list of organizations that actively support healthy school meals and nutrition education.

The remainder of this chapter is devoted to providing practical, hands-on ideas for improving the school nutrition environment on a local level.

Table 12-1

Healthy School Nutrition Environment: Checklist For Success

Are you making the grade when it comes to a healthy school nutrition environment? Rate your efforts and see for yourself:

_____1. Do your menus meet the nutrition standards of the 2010 Dietary Guidelines for Americans and *MyPlate*? (3=absolutely; 2=they could use some improvement; 1=not really)

_____2. Do your menus take into consideration student preferences and offer a variety of choices that appeal to various ethnic groups in your school? (3=absolutely; 2=they could use some improvement; 1=not really)

_____3. Do you offer students a positive eating environment with adequate time to eat? (3=yes, at a majority of schools in the district; 2=at some schools; 1=not really)

_____4. Has your school or district implemented a local school wellness policy that promotes healthful eating? (3=yes; 2=it's in development; 1=no)

_____5. Is there a comprehensive nutrition education curriculum in place in your district? (3=yes; 2=it's in development; 1=no)

_____6. Is the school nutrition department integrated with classroom nutrition education? (3=yes, we work on several programs and activities; 2=somewhat, on occasion at some schools; 1=no)

_____7. Is there a competitive food policy in place that prohibits the direct competition of minimally nutritious foods with the school meal program? (3=yes; 2=it's in development; 1=no)

_____8. Do you provide your staff with ongoing inservice training in nutrition and personal wellness? (3=yes; 2=only occasionally; 1=no)

_____9. Are family members and the community involved in supporting and reinforcing nutrition education? Do you reach out to parents and other adults with your nutrition education efforts? (3=yes, frequently; 2=only occasionally; 1=rarely)

_____10. Do you have an evaluation component in place to measure your progress in reaching nutrition education goals? (3=yes, for all our efforts; 2=only on some programs; 1=no)

How did you do? If you got a perfect score of 30, congratulations! Share your ideas and success stories with colleagues from other districts. If you scored 15 or higher, you are making progress. Keep up the good work and don't get discouraged. If you scored below 15, don't despair! Start by taking just one or two categories and really concentrating your efforts in these areas over the next year.

Adapted from: Evers C. (2000) A nutrition education report card. School Foodservice & Nutrition. June/July:22-30.

Table 12-2

Resources for Healthier Schools

Let's Move!
www.letsmove.gov
In February 2010, First Lady Michelle Obama launched Let's Move!, a comprehensive initiative involving multiple stakeholders, to solve the problem of childhood obesity in a generation.

Chefs Move to Schools
www.chefsmovetoschools.org
The Chefs Move to Schools program is part of the Let's Move! initiative. The program pairs chefs with schools in their communities with the goal of educating kids about food and proper nutrition. Chefs also partner with school nutrition staff, teachers and administrators.

The HealthierUS School Challenge
www.fns.usda.gov/tn/healthierus/index.html
The HealthierUS School Challenge is an initiative established to recognize those schools participating in the National School Lunch Program that have created healthier school environments through promotion of nutrition and physical activity.

Action for Healthy Kids (AHK)
www.actionforhealthykids.org
Action for Healthy Kids serves schools in every state with expertise, volunteers, a rich database of information and programs and services. AHK helps schools develop and implement an action plan, including a local school wellness policy, to improve nutrition and physical activity.

Alliance for a Healthier Generation
www.healthiergeneration.org
The Alliance for a Healthier Generation is a joint venture between the American Heart Association and Clinton Foundation. The Alliance's Healthy Schools Program supports more than 14,000 U.S. schools in creating environments that promote physical activity and healthy eating.

Fuel Up to Play 60 (FUTP60)
www.fueluptoplay60.com
FUTP60 is a school-based nutrition and physical activity program founded by the National Dairy Council and the National Football League. Students and adults work together to select and implement a series of "Plays" that result in long-term changes.

Healthy Kids Challenge (HKC)
www.healthykidschallenge.com
HKC is a nonprofit organization that helps school, community, business and health leaders take action for kids to eat, move and enjoy a healthy balance. Created by registered dietitians, HKC offers solutions through workshops, events, toolkits, a website, newsletters and programming.

Nutrition in the Cafeteria

IMPLEMENTING THE DIETARY GUIDELINES

Using the Dietary Guidelines for Americans to plan and prepare school meals is not difficult, especially if changes are made gradually. Involving students in the process is more likely to result in a successful transition (see "Ask the Students" section below). Technical assistance is available to programs seeking healthful changes. Child Nutrition personnel at the state level can often serve as technical consultants and trainers for schools implementing healthier menus and nutrition education programs. Appendix B lists organizations that provide school nutrition professionals with menus, recipes and other resources useful in implementing the dietary guidelines.

School meal programs throughout the country are as diverse and varied as the individuals they serve. But in spite of cultural, geographic and ethnic differences, all schools can succeed at making the cafeteria a healthful environment. Table 12-3 lists easy-to implement changes that make a big nutritional difference in the menu.

OFFER CHOICE & VARIETY

From clothing to entertainment to careers, today's children have a multitude of choices compared to previous generations. The same is true for food — children definitely want a say in what they eat.

Schools can devise a system of variety and choice that improves nutrition habits and reduces waste. A number of school districts have successfully implemented this type of system at the elementary level, offering a choice of three or more entrées and self-serve variety bars which feature a wide selection of fruits, vegetables and whole grains.

One Oregon school (North Plains Elementary) witnessed particularly dramatic changes after the implementation of the choice system. Average daily lunch participation increased from 61 percent to 73 percent, the produce order jumped from 40 to 100 pounds per week and the amount of

Table 12-3

15 Steps Toward Healthier School Meals

1. Use fat-free yogurt as the base for fruit and vegetable dips, salad dressings and breakfast toppings. Yogurt adds calcium, protein and other nutrients.

2. Substitute reduced-fat mayonnaise for the full-fat variety.

3. Increase the fiber in baked products by using whole grain flour. If acceptance is a problem, begin by using a 50-50 blend of whole grain and white flour. Adding wheat germ, bran or flaxseed to baked goods also increases nutrients and fiber.

4. Offer whole grains such as brown and wild rice, quinoa and whole grain pasta.

5. Offer several fruit and vegetable choices daily. Purchase canned fruits packed in water or fruit juice. Lightly steam vegetables to preserve quality and nutrients.

6. Use part-skim mozzarella on pizza, in Mexican dishes and sliced for sandwiches. Test reduced-fat and reduced-sodium cheddar and American to find brands that are acceptable in taste and texture.

7. Reduce the amount of butter used in cooking. If possible, switch to a soft vegetable spread that is 100% free of trans fat (see page 88).

8. When serving pizza, use a whole grain crust and always offer at least one vegetarian choice. Experiment with new vegetable combinations such as pepper rings, broccoli florets, shredded carrots or chopped spinach. Layer vegetables on top of sauce, then cover with cheese.

9. Use the leanest ground meat available, whether lean beef or turkey. Drain after browning and rinse with hot water to remove more fat.

10. Plant flowers in the deep fryer! Prepare foods by baking, broiling or steaming.

11. Remove salt shakers from lunchroom tables.

12. Offer breakfast items that are high in fiber and low in sugar, such as whole grain English muffins, whole grain bagels, low-sugar cold cereals and whole-wheat toast. Purchase reduced-sugar syrup for pancakes and waffles.

13. Write purchasing specifications with nutrition in mind. Clearly state the upper limits of fat, sodium, sugar, etc. that you define as acceptable in a particular product. Insist that nutritionally modified products meet taste and quality standards.

14. Work with manufacturers to develop and offer nutritious products that are acceptable to children. Offer to test and evaluate new items in your program.

15. Work with local farmers to implement a farm-to-school program that highlights locally grown produce, milk, beans, meat and other commodities. The USDA offers assistance on Farm to School initiatives at www.fns.usda.gov/cnd/F2S

food left uneaten on the average tray dropped 47 percent. By keeping an eye on the garbage cans and adjusting production accordingly, the school actually saw the average food cost per meal drop 16 percent. Because students were selecting much of their lunches, serving time was ultimately reduced (once children got used to the new system) and labor costs held steady.

A cafeteria that features variety and choice also provides options for children who are vegetarian, have specific ethnic preferences or have medical conditions such as diabetes, food allergies, lactose intolerance, or celiac disease or gluten intolerance.

Research from the Cornell Center for Behavioral Economics in Child Nutrition Program supports offering choice in schools. Their *Smarter Lunchroom Movement* focuses on the behavioral and environmental changes that can lead a student to unknowingly make healthier lunch choices without knowing they were "nudged" in that direction. Lunchroom design as well as behavioral cues are a centerpiece of their research. A few examples of the *Smarter Lunchroom Movement* are highlighted in Table 12-4.

ASK THE STUDENTS!

When making menu changes, the best "consultants" you can obtain are free and readily available — they are the students you serve each day. When kids feel ownership in the meal program, they are more likely to support and patronize school breakfast and lunch. Revamping the menu without the students' knowledge or support can drive students away from the school meal program.

Since food becomes nutrition only after it is eaten, menu changes should reflect students' food preferences. One way to elicit this information is to form student advisory groups. Some schools refer to these as Nutrition Advisory Councils (NACs).

Education is the key to making advisory councils work effectively. Students should first gain a clear understanding of the goals of the school meal program, which are to provide nutritious meals that are acceptable to

Table 12-4

Lessons from Smarter Lunchrooms

Q. Would you like fruit with your lunch?

A. According to research from the Cornell Center for Behavioral Economics in Child Nutrition Program, asking this simple question in the school lunchroom can have a big impact on how much fruit kids take and eat. Offering two choices of a fruit or vegetable is even better. Kids given a choice between carrots and celery **ate** 91% of the vegetable taken vs. 69% when carrots alone were offered.

This is just one example of the research conducted by the *Smarter Lunchroom Movement.* Director Brian Wansink, Ph.D. is a food psychology pioneer and author of the bestselling book, *Mindless Eating: Why We Eat More Than We Think* (Bantam, 2010).

While many of the principles of the smarter lunchroom may seem like common sense, the team at Cornell employs scientific methodology to find the most effective ways to steer kids towards more nutritious choices at school. Among their findings:

Offer choices
Schools sometimes attempt to eliminate all but the most healthy food choices. This is a mistake. When kids feel that nutrition is forced upon them, rebellion is the predictable outcome. Instead, offer a wider variety of healthier foods (more fruit, vegetables, low-fat dairy and whole grain choices) while limiting the number and variety of less-healthy choices.

Keep healthy food up front and center
Moving the salad bar from a cafeteria wall to the center of the cafeteria results in a 200-300% increase in daily salad sales. Likewise, putting more nutritious lunch choices at the beginning of the line prompts students to make healthier choices.

Make it look good
Instead of hiding fruit behind a stainless steel counter, place it in a colorful fruit bowl. Attractive, visible and accessible merchandising of sandwiches, yogurt, salads and other better-for-you choices ups the odds that they will land on the lunch tray.

Give foods fun, catchy names
In one cafeteria, when the same "bean burrito" was renamed "Big Bad Bean Burrito," sales shot up by more than 40%. Sales of carrots doubled when they were renamed "X-Ray Vision Carrots."

Learn more at www.smarterlunchrooms.org

students and to operate the program in a cost-effective manner. Ideally, students selected for the council will have some basic understanding of nutrition and why it is important. If not, this may be an ideal forum for hands-on nutrition education activities.

Children can also gain skills in constructive criticism and problem solving. Some students may be reluctant to offer feedback, while others may present a very negative picture of the school cafeteria (we've all heard the jokes and negative comments). A sample dialogue that I have used successfully with students is included in Table 12-5.

Role of the Advisory Council The advisory council can participate in the school meal program in a variety of ways. Examples of NAC activities are outlined below.

▲ Poll the student body to find out the most- and least-liked favorite foods served at school. Brainstorm ways that favorite foods can be modified to meet the Dietary Guidelines for Americans.

▲ Conduct plate waste studies to determine which foods are consistently thrown out, uneaten (see Chapter 7, page 113 for an example).

▲ Taste test and evaluate new recipes, commodities or vendor food items that have been nutritionally "improved" (e.g., reduced in fat, sodium or sugar, whole grain flour substituted for white, fortified with calcium, etc.).

▲ Plan a menu once a month, designating it as "NAC" day. To give students real-world experience, teach them to cost out the menu and perform a nutritional analysis of their chosen meal, making adjustments as needed.

▲ Train advisory council members as peer educators. Provide them with simple lesson ideas that they can teach in classrooms around the school. Suggest they develop and perform a noontime skit on good nutrition for the student body (see Chapter 9 for ideas).

▲ Enlist the advisory council's help in devising a marketing plan. Involve members in the development of a cafeteria slogan, logo, mascot or catchy name.

Table 12-5

Teaching Constructive Criticism

Students, particularly those in the intermediate grades, may resort to negative remarks when describing the food served at school. Responding to students in a defensive and critical manner only serves to worsen the situation. Below is a sample dialogue that illustrates how to defuse the situation and promote co-operative problem solving.

LEADER: Would anyone like to share their thoughts about the school breakfast or lunch program?

STUDENT 1: It's so-o-o-o-o gross!

STUDENT 2: Yeah, I wouldn't feed that nasty junk to my dog!

LEADER: What I think I'm hearing is that some of you dislike the food served in the cafeteria. The problem is, I haven't heard much useful information so far. Right now, if I were to sit down and plan next month's menu, the comments I just heard sure wouldn't help me much.

STUDENT 3: I have a complaint — sometimes when I eat the third lunch period, the milk has been sitting out for a while and it's warm.

LEADER: Thank you. It helps when you give me a specific example of a problem that you see in the cafeteria. You have a valid point — milk should not sit at room temperature for that length of time. Do any of you have suggestions on how to solve this problem?

STUDENT 4: Maybe you could keep cartons of milk in a bowl filled with ice.

STUDENT 5: How about using one of those refrigerators that can be rolled into the cafeteria at lunchtime?

LEADER: Those are great suggestions, students. In fact, I'm going to start a list of your ideas that I can use in my planning.

STUDENT 1: Do you think you could do something so that the broccoli isn't mushy? My mom always serves it raw with ranch dip. I like it that way.

STUDENT 2: And I wish we could have a salad bar more often. I always eat lunch the days we have a salad bar.

LEADER: Thank you, students. It is very helpful when you give specific examples and useful suggestions. With your help, I can make changes that improve the program for everyone.

▲ Give the advisory council space on the menu for a "student's corner" where they can provide tips about nutrition and facts about the school meal program.

▲ Be sure to acknowledge and reward the work of the advisory council. Award students with special privileges, certificates or prizes such as pencils, notepads, stickers, water bottles or movie passes.

COMPETITIVE FOODS — TAKING A STAND

Competitive food sales undermine nutrition and health goals. When a child can choose between a candy bar from the school store or a healthy lunch in the cafeteria, too often the candy bar will win out.

The issue of competitive foods is complex, often evoking debate among school nutrition providers, administrators and even parent groups. In times of stretched budgets, school groups, athletic teams and administrators resort to the sale of candy, pop, fried chips, cookies and other empty calorie foods — often through vending machines — to boost revenues.

While some states and school districts have official policies banning or restricting competitive foods, many schools choose to ignore the issue, fearful of losing the revenue that supports school programs. Clearly, creative solutions for funding important programs are needed. We can no longer afford to balance budgets at the expense of children's health.

Unpopular as the issue may be, it is important to highlight the competitive food issue in each school. Offering healthful alternatives for fundraisers, stocking vending machines with more nutritious food and beverage choices and limiting student store sales to nutritious foods are all positive steps to creating a healthier school environment.

At the very least, a compromise should be agreed on and enforced that limits the sale of empty calorie foods to after school or during sporting or extracurricular events.

Cafeteria Atmosphere

▨ FROM DRAB TO DELIGHTFUL

With effort and creativity, the school cafeteria can become a bright and cheery place to eat. Some ideas:

▲ Paint can do wonders for the cafeteria. Replace drab, boring walls with blocks of bright colors. Or invite the art teacher or a guest artist to coordinate students in the design and painting of a colorful cafeteria mural. (A food and fitness theme would be especially nice!)

▲ Collect and frame colorful posters of food to display near the serving areas. Many of the food companies and commissions listed in Appendix B provide free posters and other materials for display.

▲ Encourage students to design posters for the cafeteria that depict good nutrition themes.

▲ Display a "nutrition corner" bulletin board that is changed regularly throughout the year. Examples of themes include *MyPlate*, food and fitness, how food promotes a healthy heart, how to read the *Nutrition Facts* food label, the importance of calcium in building strong bones, how breakfast fuels learning and facts about the school meal program. Consider a nearby table with handout information for students, staff and parents. Teachers, students and school nutrition staff can work cooperatively to design and maintain the bulletin board throughout the year.

▲ Add a personal touch to the cafeteria: Spruce up the serving line with colorful garnishes, display bright vinyl tablecloths on serving tables (fabric stores are an inexpensive source of colorful vinyl), purchase or make eye-catching aprons for nutrition staff and student assistants or occasionally put out fresh cut flowers on cafeteria tables.

TIME TO EAT

Offering tasty, nutritious food in a pleasant environment is not enough, though — children must have time to eat. It sounds simple enough, yet schools pressed for instructional time frequently shortchange kids by skimping on lunch time. Shortened lunch periods, coupled with long lines and slow service, may give children as few as five minutes to eat! In some schools, students opt for sack lunches just so they can bypass the lunch line.

From the time children sit down with their tray, they should be guaranteed a minimum of 20 uninterrupted minutes to eat. More time may be required for students with certain disabilities. The same holds true for breakfast — bus and morning schedules should be adjusted to allow ample time for children eating breakfast at school.

Marketing & Education

TOOT YOUR HORN!

Many school nutrition operators would do well to boast more, spreading the good news about their programs. Students, teachers and parents may not know, for instance, that the "chicken nuggets" printed on the menu are actually a baked product made from minimally processed whole chicken or that the dinner rolls contain 50 percent whole-wheat flour or that a fruit and vegetable bar is available daily. Parents, the media and the community may be unaware of point-of-choice nutrition information in the cafeteria, local produce served during "harvest of the month" events or classroom nutrition lessons taught by nutrition staff.

> **Check this out:**
> Registered dietitian and school nutrition advocate Dayle Hayes founded *School Meals That Rock*, a place to share and celebrate what is right with school nutrition in America. Hayes frequently updates her page with examples of colorful, nutritious and delicious school meals served in school districts throughout the nation.
> www.facebook.com/SchoolMealsThatRock

Effectively communicating your message is an essential ingredient to marketing success. The first step is to define your target markets. This could include the children you serve, school personnel (teachers, staff, administrators) or the community (parents, school board, media). Next, devise ways to reach these groups with your message. The examples below highlight techniques for publicizing the school meal program.

▲ Start with the menu. An already familiar piece, the menu adorns thousands of refrigerators each month throughout your school community. Reserve space on the front of the menu for nutrition tidbits, program highlights and announcements of special promotions. Use words and phrases that denote nutrition to describe foods offered on menus, such as "whole-grain" rolls, "low-fat" dressing, "garden fresh" broccoli florets or "Teriyaki chicken bowl with vegetables and brown rice."

Think about the design of the menu, too. Avoid using the same standard format month after month. Enlist the help of school staff (art teachers or district graphic designers) to enhance the design of the menu. Work with a web designer to make sure the online version of the menu is eye-catching, informative and interactive.

▲ Become an integral part of the school environment. School nutrition staff should take a keen interest in the events and programs in their school. Participate in monthly staff meetings and regularly contribute recipes, nutrition updates and other items to the school newsletter, website and facebook page. Volunteer to assist teachers with food and nutrition lesson planning.

▲ Be proactive by inviting parents, the school board or the media to eat school breakfast or lunch. Highlight the nutrition messages and healthful choices served each day in the cafeteria. Send out notices of special promotions, contests and events.

Don't let media coverage about the downside of school meals mar your program. Prepare a fact sheet that highlights your mission, statistics about those you serve and a summary of positive outcomes. Send a press release to local media that emphasizes how your program offers healthful choices as well as nutrition education.

BECOME A PARTNER IN EDUCATION

The nutrition concepts taught in the classroom can effectively be reinforced in the cafeteria. Beyond a health-promoting menu, school nutrition providers can also participate in nutrition education through a variety of practices, activities and promotions:

▲ **Merchandise Healthful Foods:** Make sure healthful food choices beg to be eaten. The use of baskets, attractive arrangements, colorful food choices and garnishes will make nutritious foods stand out.

▲ **Point-of-Choice Nutrition Information:** Display a simple nutrition analysis of foods commonly served in the cafeteria. (Consider working with a fourth or fifth grade class on determining and displaying the information.)

Include the analysis for calories, fat, carbohydrate, protein, fiber and sodium. Especially meaningful are comparisons of different forms of the same food such as a vegetarian versus a pepperoni pizza.

Consider highlighting other nutrients from time to time, complemented by informative posters, bulletin boards and handouts. Examples include iron, potassium, fiber, zinc, B vitamins or calcium.

▲ **100 Percent Participation:** You can achieve complete participation — one classroom at a time, that is. Once a month, set up a "make your own lunch" bar in a chosen classroom. Students will learn basic food

> **Everyone in school nutrition is a Nutrition Educator!**
>
> Attention school nutrition staff! Have you ever:
>
> - Nudged the fruit basket to the front of the counter so more students would be tempted to grab a piece?
> - Put up eye-catching signage to promote a new healthful entrée or the local "harvest of the month" veggie?
> - Greeted a student with, "See you at breakfast tomorrow"?
> - Artfully arranged the salad bar to make it more enticing to students?
>
> If you answered "yes" to any of the above, you are promoting good nutrition habits. Whether or not it's apparent, everyone who works in the school cafeteria also wears the title of nutrition educator.

preparation skills as they assemble their own meals. Food bars that work particularly well include a setup for sub or pita pocket sandwiches, chef salads, French bread pizza topped with vegetables or healthy tostados (made from whole corn tortillas, various beans, lean ground beef or ground turkey, low-fat cheese, salsa, olives, tomatoes, peppers, avocados, onions and a yogurt-based sauce). Cover and label each student's lunch to be passed out when they come through the serving line. Or, as time permits, coordinate the activity right before their scheduled lunch period and allow students to eat in their classroom.

If possible, make a lunch date with each classroom in the school over the course of the year. Besides being a great opportunity for nutrition education, this activity is also a powerful way to market the school meal program to students.

▲ **Promotions and Events:** Make the cafeteria a fun place to learn with special promotions and thematic menus. "New Food Days" or "Food of the Week" events can feature small incentives for students who select a new nutritious food item. Menu, recipe or poster contests, nutrition bingo cards and breakfast ticket raffles are all fun ways to teach nutrition and promote the school meal program.

Posters, suggested menus and other resources are available for specific events such as National School Breakfast and Lunch Weeks (available through the *School Nutrition Association*) or National Nutrition Month (sponsored by the *Academy of Nutrition and Dietetics*). There are also a multitude of other special holidays and months, celebrating everything from grandparents to pickles to potatoes to heart health!

▲ **Teaching Students:** Many of the suggested nutrition activities and lessons described in Chapters 4–11 could easily be presented by school food and nutrition professionals. Nearly every chapter includes lesson ideas that interface with the cafeteria (identified by the cafeteria icon).

Inviting classes to tour the school or central kitchen is a memorable way to introduce students to the school nutrition operation. To enhance the experience, combine the tour with a brief lesson on nutrition, give students the opportunity to plan a menu, set up a taste test for a new product or challenge students to find a food from each food group during the tour.

School nutrition staff can also assist in career education, highlighting the job requirements and tasks of jobs such as cook, baker, chef, truck driver, school nutrition director, registered dietitian or food technologist.

Appendix A
Guidelines for Safe Classroom Cooking

"I liked how you served the food with your gloves. My Mom asked if anyone touched the food." —Jenny

With so many hands busy at work, classroom cooking poses a challenge for keeping food sanitary and working conditions safe. When planning cooking projects, be sure to enlist the help of school staff or parent volunteers. The reminders below are essential for a safe, enjoyable cooking experience.

BEFORE YOU BEGIN

▲ Send a letter home to parents explaining that the class will periodically participate in cooking projects that enhance the curriculum. *Be sure to elicit information on food allergies or intolerances or any specific medical conditions that prohibit their children from eating certain foods.* Include permission slips for parents to sign and return.

▲ Call the local health department to find out how to become certified as a food handler. You may be required to take a course or pass a test before handling food in a public setting (local and state regulations vary).

▲ Be sure that all staff and volunteers who assist with classroom cooking have read and understand the guidelines presented here.

PROPER HANDWASHING IS VITAL!

▲ Demonstrate to students the techniques for proper handwashing. Thoroughly scrub all surfaces of the hands and nails with soap, rinse with warm water and dry with clean paper towels.

▲ The factor most important in producing clean hands is time. Encourage students to scrub hands for the duration of the "A-B-C song" (about 20 seconds).

FIGHT BAC!
Fight BAC is a great resource from the Partnership for Food Safety Education, addressing the core four steps to food safety: Clean, Separate, Cook and Chill. Download and order materials for classroom food safety education at: www.fightbac.org

▲ If the restroom is used for handwashing prior to handling food, prop the door open. Otherwise, students will touch the bacteria-covered doorknob on their way out.

▲ Remind students to wash hands after using the restroom; touching their faces, hair or neighbor; blowing their noses or sneezing; and after handling raw meat, chicken, eggs or fish.

Tie in the concept of handwashing with a science lesson about bacteria and viruses. There are kits available that utilize an ultraviolet light and special soap to reveal whether hands contain "germs" (similar to the way dental disclosing tablets reveal the presence of plaque on teeth). The following companies sell a variety of kits and products:

   ♦ Glo Germ, available at www.glogerm.com

   ♦ Germ Juice, available at www.germjuice.com

   ♦ Glitterbug, available at www.glitterbug.com

Another germ-based science activity is to culture various surfaces such as hands, tables or doorknobs and grow on a nutrient-rich medium in a petri dish. Once the experiment is completed, petri dishes should be rinsed with a bleach solution and disposed of properly.

PROVIDE A SANITARY WORK SURFACE FOR HANDLING FOOD

▲ Desks or tables should be cleared, cleaned and covered with clean butcher paper or a vinyl placemat or tablecloth. Cutting boards should be cleaned with hot, soapy water and a sanitizing solution such as diluted bleach. (To make the bleach solution, mix 1 tablespoon institutional-strength bleach or 2 tablespoons household bleach into one gallon of water.)

▲ Designate one knife and cutting board for raw produce. Avoid cross contamination with protein-based foods.

▲ Wash and sanitize all work surfaces, cutting boards and utensils after they have come into contact with raw meat, fish, poultry or eggs.

EMPHASIZE SAFETY WITH KNIVES AND EQUIPMENT

▲ Before allowing children to begin work on food projects, demonstrate the proper use of knives and equipment such as graters, cheese slicers and can openers. Advise students to always cut toward their work surface and away from their hands.

▲ Any equipment, even plastic serrated knives, plastic chopsticks, toothpicks or wooden skewers, can be dangerous if handled improperly. Promptly remove students who are behaving in a reckless manner with tools or equipment.

▲ Always use two dry potholders when removing foods from the microwave or oven. Be sure to turn off the stove, oven, electric fry pan, etc. when you are done cooking. Avoid knocking hot pots off the stove by turning pot and pan handles inward.

ORGANIZING COOKING PROJECTS

▲ For projects that students will prepare individually at their desks, assign three or four adult volunteers and/or students to hand out food and utensils. Those passing out supplies should practice good hygiene and always wear clean disposable gloves.

▲ One way to efficiently run a classroom cooking project is to organize an assembly line. Using a long table, line up the ingredients for such items as mini-bagel pizzas, rolled burritos, stuffed pita sandwiches or fruit-yogurt parfaits. If you utilize this method, make sure there is at least one adult at both the beginning and end of the line. Just before starting through the line, students should put on clean disposable gloves.

▲ Time your projects so that foods do not sit at room temperature for more than two hours. The "danger zone" for rapid bacterial growth is between 40 and 140 degrees Fahrenheit (i.e., room temperature). Pick up foods from the kitchen right before you begin the project and return leftovers upon completion. Do not allow students to save perishable foods to eat later in the day.

▲ Don't sample food products prepared with raw eggs. Even one tasty spoonful of cookie batter could harbor dangerous bacteria. Recipes that call for raw eggs, such as eggnog or homemade ice cream, should use an egg substitute that has been pasteurized.

NOTE: The guidelines presented here pertain to children of elementary school age (ages 5 to 12). When conducting projects with younger children, avoid foods that could lodge in the throat such as whole grapes, popcorn, peanut butter, nuts and hard pieces of fruit or vegetable.

Appendix B
Selected Resources

Note: Some companies and organizations are listed under more than one heading.

Audiovisual/Education Resource Catalogs

The following companies feature a wide variety of resources including books, DVDs, music, posters, computer software, food models and other teaching tools.

Food and Health Communications
  800-462-2352
  www.foodandhealth.com

FoodPlay Productions
  800-FOODPLAY
  www.foodplay.com

Health Edco/WRS Group
  800-299-3366
  www.healthedco.com

Learning Zone Express
  888-455-7003
  www.learningzonexpress.com

MacGill Discount School Nurse Supplies
  800-323-2841
  www.macgill.com

NASCO Nutrition Teaching Aids Catalog
  800-558-9595
  www.enasco.com

NCES (Nutrition, Counseling and Education Services)
  877-623-7266
  www.ncescatalog.com

NEAT Solutions for Healthy Children
888-577-NEAT
www.neatsolutions.com

School Health Corporation
866-323-5465
www.schoolhealth.com

School Nurse Supply, Inc.
800-485-2737
schoolnursesupplyinc.com

The OrganWise Guys
800-786-1730
www.organwiseguys.com

Yummy Designs
888-74-YUMMY
www.yummydesigns.com

Books for Children

See index entry "Books, Children" for a list of all children's books referenced throughout this book (coded by reading level).

Cookbooks for Kids

Amico, J. & Drummond, K. (2005). *The coming to America cookbook : Delicious recipes and fascinating stories from America's many cultures.* Hoboken, N.J: Wiley.

Cook, D. (2008). *The kids' multicultural cookbook : food & fun from around the world.* Nashville, Tenn: Williamson Books.

Dodge, A. (2008). *Around the world cookbook.* New York: DK Publishing.

Katzen, M. (2005). *Salad people and more real recipes: a new cookbook for preschoolers & up.* Berkeley, Calif: Tricycle Press.

Negrin, J. (2010). *Easy meals to cook with kids: healthy, family-friendly recipes from around the world.* S.l: Authorhouse.

Fitness

Let's Move!
   www.letsmove.gov

National Association for Sport and Physical Education
   www.aahperd.org/naspe

NFL Play 60
   www.nflrush.com/play60

Physical Activity Tracker (one component of the *MyPlate* SuperTracker)
   www.choosemyplate.gov/SuperTracker

President's Council on Fitness, Sports & Nutrition
   www.fitness.gov

The President's Challenge
   www.presidentschallenge.org

The Truth on Health
   Boston Celtics Captain Paul Pierce founded this site to promote kid's
   fitness and health. Connie Evers contributes guest nutrition blogs.
   www.truthonhealth.org

Hopper, C., Fisher, B., & Munoz, K. (2008). *Physical activity and nutrition
   for health*. Champaign, IL: Human Kinetics.

Food Companies/Commissions

Food companies and commissions can be a useful source for posters, flyers, recipes, nutrition information and nutrition education curricula.

A word of caution: Please read all company sponsored materials carefully
before using with students. Some materials may contain biased information. Choose materials that present a balanced view of nutrition.

Dairy Council of California
   www.dairycouncilofca.org

California Kiwi Fruit Commission
   www.kiwifruit.org

California Strawberry Commission
www.calstrawberry.com

California Table Grape Commission
www.tablegrape.com

Canned Food Alliance
www.mealtime.org

Dole Food Company
www.dole.com

Florida Department of Citrus
www.floridajuice.com

Grain Foods Foundation
www.gowiththegrain.org

International Food Information Council (IFIC) Foundation
www.foodinsight.org

National Dairy Council
www.nationaldairycouncil.org

Oregon Dairy Council/Nutrition Education Services
www.oregondairycouncil.org

Oregon Raspberry & Blackberry Commission
www.oregon-berries.com

Produce for Better Health Foundation
www.fruitsandveggiesmorematters.org

The Peanut Institute
www.peanut-institute.org

United States Potato Board
www.uspotatoes.com

USA Pears
www.usapears.com

Washington State Apple Commission
www.bestapples.com

Washington State Dairy Council
www.eatsmart.org

Washington State Fruit Commission/Northwest Cherries
www.nwcherries.com

Wheat Foods Council
www.wheatfoods.org

Gardening

School Gardening Resource Site from USDA
healthymeals.nal.usda.gov/hsmrs/garden

The edible schoolyard project
www.edibleschoolyard.org

Garden ABCs
www.GardenABCs.com

Farm to School
www.farmtoschool.org

Kids Gardening
www.kidsgardening.com

Life Lab
www.lifelab.org

Lovejoy, S. (1999). Roots, shoots, buckets & boots: gardening together
with children. New York: Workman Pub.

Patten, E. (2003). Healthy foods from healthy soils: a hands-on resource
for educators. Gardner, Me: Tilbury House Publishers.

People's Garden from USDA
www.usda.gov/peoplesgarden

General Reference

Duyff, R. (2012). *American Dietetic Association complete food and nutrition guide.* Hoboken, N.J.: Wiley.

Kobuszewski, A. (2011). *Food, field to fork: how to grow sustainably, shop wisely, cook nutritiously, and eat deliciously.* San Leandro, CA: AnitaBeHealthy Publishing.

Shanley, E. & Thompson, C. (2011). *Fueling the teen machine : what it takes to make good choices for yourself every day.* Boulder, Colo: Bull Pub.

Shield, J. & Mullen, M. (2011). *Healthy eating, healthy weight for kids and teens.* Chicago, IL: Academy of Nutrition and Dietetics.

Sizer, F. & Whitney, E. (2012). *Nutrition Concepts and Controversies, My-Plate Update.* Brooks/Cole Pub Co.

Government

Centers for Disease Control and Prevention (CDC)
www.cdc.gov

Dietary Guidelines for Americans, 2010
www.cnpp.usda.gov/dietaryguidelines.htm

Food Labeling and Nutrition
U.S. Food and Drug Administration

Food and Nutrition Information Center (FNIC)
fnic.nal.usda.gov

Food Safety
foodsafety.gov

Fruits and Veggies Matter
www.fruitsandveggiesmatter.gov

Healthier US School Challenge
www.fns.usda.gov/tn/healthierus/index.html

Let's Move!
www.letsmove.gov

MyPlate Food Guide
www.choosemyplate.gov

National Institute of Health , Heart, Lung, and Blood Institute
wecan.nhlbi.nih.gov

National Institute of Health , Office of Dietary Supplements
ods.od.nih.gov/

Nutrition
nutrition.gov

People's Garden from USDA
www.usda.gov/peoplesgarden

President's Council on Fitness, Sports & Nutrition
www.fitness.gov

Team Nutrition
teamnutrition.usda.gov

U.S. Food and Drug Administration Nutrition Facts Label Program
www.fda.gov/Food/ResourcesForYou/Consumers/NFLPM/default.htm

USDA Agriculture in the Classroom
www.agclassroom.org

USDA Center for Nutrition Policy and Promotion
www.usda.gov/cnpp

USDA Food and Nutrition Service Farm to School Initiative
www.fns.usda.gov/cnd/f2s/

USDA Nutrition Evidence Library
www.nel.gov

Organizations

Academy of Nutrition and Dietetics
www.eatright.org

Action for Healthy Kids
www.actionforhealthykids.org

Alliance for a Healthier Generation
www.healthiergeneration.org

American Diabetes Association
www.diabetes.org

American Heart Association
www.heart.org

American Institute for Cancer Research
www.aicr.org

California Foundation for Agriculture in the Classroom
www.cfaitc.org

Celiac Disease Foundation
www.celiac.org

Center for Science in the Public Interest
www.cspinet.org

School Nutrition Association
www.schoolnutrition.org

Food Research and Action Center
www.frac.org

Society for Nutrition Education and Behavior
www.sne.org

The Food Allergy & Anaphylaxis Network
www.foodallergy.org

The Robert Wood Johnson Foundation
rwjf.org

The Vegetarian Resource Group
www.vrg.org

School Nutrition

Action for Healthy Kids
www.actionforhealthykids.org

Alliance for a Healthier Generation
www.healthiergeneration.org

Breakfast in the Classroom
www.breakfastintheclassroom.org

Chefs Move to Schools
www.chefsmovetoschools.org

Fuel Up to Play 60 (FUTP60)
www.fueluptoplay60.com

Harvest of the Month, Network for a Healthy California
www.harvestofthemonth.cdph.ca.gov

Healthy Kids Challenge
www.healthykidschallenge.com

National Food Service Management Institute
www.nfsmi.org

National Farm to School Network
www.farmtoschool.org

School Nutrition Association
www.schoolnutrition.org

School Nutrition Services, A Practice Group of the Academy of Nutrition and Dietetics www.snsdpg.org

Smarter Lunchrooms Movement
smarterlunchrooms.org

Start Smart Eating and Reading
extension.oregonstate.edu/catalog/html/4h/4h6830/startsmart1.html

Team Nutrition
www.fns.usda.gov/tn

The HealthierUS School Challenge
www.fns.usda.gov/tn/healthierus/index.html

USDA Food and Nutrition Service Farm to School Initiative
www.fns.usda.gov/cnd/f2s/

Web Sites

Children's Nutrition Research Center - Baylor College of Medicine
kidsnutrition.org

FOOD: Nutrition, Safety & Cooking, UNL Extension in Lancaster County
lancaster.unl.edu/food/

Fruit & Veggies More Matters
www.fruitsandveggiesmorematters.org/

Iowa State Extension Food Safety Project
www.extension.iastate.edu/foodsafety/

Kids Eat Right
www.kidseatright.org

National Association of Anorexia Nervosa and Associated Eating Disorders
www.anad.org

Nourish Interactive
www.nourishinteractive.com

Nutrition Blog Network (blogs by registered dietitians)
nutritionblognetwork.com

Nutrition for Kids
www.nutritionforkids.com

Super Kids Nutrition
www.superkidsnutrition.com

The Food Allergy & Anaphylaxis Network
www.foodallergy.org

Web Sites for Kids

Best Bones Forever
www.bestbonesforever.gov

Body and Mind
www.bam.gov

BreakFAST & Jump To It!
www.dairycouncilofca.org/Tools/BreakFAST/

Dole Superkids
Go to www.dole.com and click on "superkids" link.

Eat Well, Play Well
www.omsi.edu/exhibits/ewpw

Food Champs
www.foodchamps.org

Kidnetic
www.kidnetic.com

KidsHealth
www.kidshealth.org

MyPlate Blastoff Game
www.fns.usda.gov/multimedia/Games/Blastoff/BlastOff_Game.html

Snacktown Smackdown
info.kp.org/richmedia/kidWisdom

Bibliography

CHAPTER 1

Alaimo, K., Olson, C., & Frongillo, E. (2001). Food insufficiency and American school-aged children's cognitive, academic, and psychosocial development. *Pediatrics*, 108(1), 44-53.

Andersen, R., Crespo, C., Bartlett, S., Cheskin, L., & Pratt, M. (1998). Relationship of physical activity and television watching with body weight and level of fatness among children: results from the Third National Health and Nutrition Examination Survey. *JAMA: The Journal of the American Medical Association*, 279(12), 938-942.

Bowman, S. (2002). Beverage choices of young females: changes and impact on nutrient intakes. *Journal of the American Dietetic Association*, 102(9), 1234-1239.

Burgess-Champoux, T., Larson, N., Neumark-Sztainer, D., Hannan, P., & Story, M. (2009). Arc family meal patterns associated with overall diet quality during the transition from early to middle adolescence? *Journal of Nutrition Education and Behavior*, 41(2), 79-86.

Centers for Disease Control and Prevention (2011). *Basics about childhood obesity*. Retrieved from http://www.cdc.gov/obesity/childhood/basics.html

Coleman-Jenson, A., Nord, M., Andrews, G., & Carlson, S. (2011). *Household food security in the united states in 2010*. Retrieved from website: http://www.ers.usda.gov/Publications/err125/

Committee on Nutrition and the Council on Sports Medicine and Fitness. (2011). Sports drinks and energy drinks for children and adolescents: Are they appropriate? *Pediatrics*, 127(6), 1182-1189. Retrieved from http://pediatrics.aappublications.org/content/127/6/1182.full

Fiorito, L., Marini, M., Francis, L., Smiciklas-Wright, H., & Birch, L. (2009). Beverage intake of girls at age 5 y predicts adiposity and weight status in childhood and adolescence. *The American Journal of Clinical Nutrition*, 90(4), 935-942.

Fiorito, L., Marini, M., Mitchell, D., Smiciklas-Wright, H., & Birch, L. (2010). Girls' early sweetened carbonated beverage intake predicts different patterns of beverage and nutrient intake across childhood and adolescence. *Journal of the American Dietetic Association*, 110(4), 543-550.

Fisher, J., Mitchell, D., Smiciklas-Wright, H., & Birch, L. (2002). Parental influences on young girls' fruit and vegetable, micronutrient, and fat intakes. *Journal of the American Dietetic Association*, 102(1), 58-64.

Foster, G., Sherman, S., Borradaile, K., Grundy, K., Vander Veur, S., Nachmani, J., & ... Shults, J. (2008). A policy-based school intervention to prevent overweight and obesity. *Pediatrics*, 121(4), e794-e802. Retrieved from http://pediatrics.aappublications.org/content/121/4/e794.full

Freedman, D., Mei, Z., Srinivasan, S., Berenson, G., & Dietz, W. (2007). Cardiovascular risk factors and excess adiposity among overweight children and adolescents: the Bogalusa Heart Study. *The Journal of Pediatrics*, 150(1), 12-17.e2.

Gillman, M., Rifas-Shiman, S., Frazier, A., Rockett, H., Camargo, C., Field, A., & ... Colditz, G. (2000). Family dinner and diet quality among older children and adolescents. *Archives of Family Medicine*, 9(3), 235-240.

Gortmaker, S., Long, D., & Yang, Y. Robert Wood Johnson Foundation, (2009). *The negative impact of sugar-sweetened beverages on children's health: A research synthesis*. Retrieved from website: http://www.rwjf.org/files/research/20091203herssb.pdf

Greer, F., & Krebs, N. (2006). Optimizing bone health and calcium intakes of infants, children, and adolescents. *Pediatrics*, 117(2), 578-585.

Harnack, L., Stang, J., & Story, M. (1999). Soft drink consumption among US children and adolescents: nutritional consequences. *Journal of the American Dietetic Association*, 99(4), 436-441.

Hartline-Grafton, H. (2011). *Food insecurity and obesity: Understanding the connections*. Food Research and Action Center. Retrieved from http://frac.org/pdf/frac_brief_understanding_the_connections.pdf

Jahns, L., Siega-Riz, A., & Popkin, B. (2001). The increasing prevalence of snacking among US children from 1977 to 1996. *The Journal of Pediatrics*, 138(4), 493-498.

Lorson, B., Melgar-Quinonez, H., & Taylor, C. (2009). Correlates of fruit and vegetable intakes in US children. *Journal of the American Dietetic Association*, 109(3), 474-478.

Ludwig, D., Peterson, K., & Gortmaker, S. (2001). Relation between consumption of sugar-sweetened drinks and childhood obesity: a prospective, observational analysis. *Lancet*, 357(9255), 505-508.

Murphy, J., Wehler, C., Pagano, M., Little, M., Kleinman, R., & Jellinek, M. (1998). Relationship between hunger and psychosocial functioning in low-income American children. *Journal of the American Academy Of Child And Adolescent Psychiatry*, 37(2), 163-170.

Nader, P., Bradley, R., Houts, R., McRitchie, M., & O'Brien, M. (2008). Moderate-to-vigorous physical activity from ages 9 to 15 years. *Journal of the American Medical Association*, 300(3), 295-305. Retrieved from http://jama.ama-assn.org/content/300/3/295.full.pdf

Nielsen, S., & Popkin, B. (2003). Patterns and trends in food portion sizes, 1977-1998. *JAMA: The Journal of the American Medical Association*, 289(4), 450-453.

Ogden, C. L., Carroll, M. D., Curtin, L. R., Lamb, L. L., & Flegal, K. M. (2010). *Prevalence of high body mass index in us children and adolescents, 2007-2008*. Retrieved from http://jama.ama-assn.org/content/303/3/242.full

Ogden, C., & Carroll, M. (2010). *Prevalence of obesity among children and adolescents: United states, trends 1963-1965 through 2007-2008.* Retrieved from http://1.usa.gov/yaKAGv

Pate, R., Mitchell , J., Byun, W., & Dowda, M. (2011). Sedentary behaviour in youth. *British Journal of Sports Medicine*, 45(11), 906-13.

Poti, J., & Popkin, B. (2011). Trends in energy intake among US children by eating location and food source, 1977-2006. *Journal of the American Dietetic Association*, 111(8), 1156-1164.

Project EAT. (n.d.). *Project results.* University of Minnesota School of Public Health. Retrieved from http://www.sph.umn.edu/epi/research/eat/results.asp

Rampersaud, G., Bailey, L., & Kauwell, G. (2003). National survey beverage consumption data for children and adolescents indicate the need to encourage a shift toward more nutritive beverages. *Journal of the American Dietetic Association*, 103(1), 97-100.

Rolls, B., Engell, D., & Birch, L. (2000). Serving portion size influences 5-year-old but not 3-year-old children's food intakes. *Journal of the American Dietetic Association*, 100(2), 232-234.

Sinha, R., Fisch, G., Teague, B., Tamborlane, W., Banyas, B., Allen, K., & ... Caprio, S. (2002). Prevalence of impaired glucose tolerance among children and adolescents with marked obesity. *The New England Journal of Medicine*, 346(11), 802-810.

Smiciklas-Wright, H., Mitchell, D., Mickle, S., Goldman, J., & Cook, A. (2003). Foods commonly eaten in the United States, 1989-1991 and 1994-1996: are portion sizes changing? *Journal of the American Dietetic Association*, 103(1), 41-47.

The President's Council on Physical Fitness and Sports. *Facts and resources on the health benefits of physical activity.* (2012). Retrieved from http://www.fitness.gov/hbpa.htm

Thomas Fungwe, P., Patricia M. Guenther, P., WenYen Juan, P., Hazel Hiza, P., & Mark Lino, P. (2009). *The quality of children's diets in 2003-04 as measured by the healthy eating index-2005.* Retrieved from http://1.usa.gov/yG9HTX

U.S. Department of Agriculture and U.S. Department of Health and Human Services. (2011). *Dietary Guidelines for Americans, 2010. 7th edition.* Retrieved from website: http://www.cnpp.usda.gov/DietaryGuidelines.htm

U.S. Department of Agriculture, Agricultural Research Service, (1999). *Food and nutrient intakes by children 1994-96, 1998.* Retrieved from website: http://1.usa.gov/wALR8U

U.S. Department of Agriculture. (2012). *ChooseMyPlate.gov Website.* Washington, DC.

U.S. Department of Agriculture. *Healthy hunger-free kids act of 2010.* Retrieved from http://www.fns.usda.gov/cnd/governance/legislation/CNR_2010.htm

U.S. Department of Education, National Center for Education Statistics, (2000). *Nutrition education in public elementary school classrooms.* NCES 2000-040. Retrieved from website: http://nces.ed.gov/pubs2000/2000040.pdf

Wansink, B., & van Ittersum, K. (2007). Portion size me: downsizing our consumption norms. *Journal of the American Dietetic Association,* 107(7), 1103-1106.

Young, L., & Nestle, M. (2002). The contribution of expanding portion sizes to the US obesity epidemic. *American Journal of Public Health,* 92(2), 246-249.

Chapter 2

Abramovitz, B., & Birch, L. (2000). Five-year-old girls' ideas about dieting are predicted by their mothers' dieting. *Journal of the American Dietetic Association*, 100(10), 1157-1163.

Basiotis, P., Lino, M., & Anand, R. USDA Center for Nutrition Policy and Promotion, (1999). *Eating breakfast greatly improves schoolchildren's diet quality*. Retrieved from website: http://1.usa.gov/xa2g1E

Borzekowski, D., & Robinson, T. (2001). The 30-second effect: an experiment revealing the impact of television commercials on food preferences of preschoolers. *Journal of the American Dietetic Association*, 101(1), 42-46.

Boyland, E., Harrold, J., Kirkham, T., Corker, C., Cuddy, J., Evans, D., & ... Halford, J. (2011). Food commercials increase preference for energy-dense foods, particularly in children who watch more television. *Pediatrics*, 128(1), e93-e100.

Byrd-Bredbenner , C., & Murray, J. (2002). A longitudinal analysis of weight and shape ideals as defined by miss america pageant winners. *Journal of the American Dietetic Association*, (S102), A-73.

Coon, K., & Tucker, K. (2002). Television and children's consumption patterns. A review of the literature. *Minerva Pediatrica*, 54(5), 423-436.

Coon, K., Goldberg, J., Rogers, B., & Tucker, K. (2001). Relationships between use of television during meals and children's food consumption patterns. *Pediatrics*, 107(1), E7.

Evers, C. (1997). Empower children to develop healthful eating habits. *Journal of the American Dietetic Association*, 97(10 Suppl 2), S116.

Field, A., Camargo, C., Taylor, C., Berkey, C., Roberts, S., & Colditz, G. (2001). Peer, parent, and media influences on the development of weight concerns and frequent dieting among preadolescent and adolescent girls and boys. *Pediatrics*, 107(1), 54-60.

Field, A., Cheung, L., Wolf, A., Herzog, D., Gortmaker, S., & Colditz, G. (1999). Exposure to the mass media and weight concerns among girls. *Pediatrics*, 103(3), E36.

Fisher, J., & Birch, L. (1999). Restricting access to palatable foods affects children's behavioral response, food selection, and intake. *The American Journal of Clinical Nutrition*, 69(6), 1264-1272.

Fisher, J., & Birch, L. (2000). Parents' restrictive feeding practices are associated with young girls' negative self-evaluation of eating. *Journal of the American Dietetic Association*, 100(11), 1341-1346.

Fisher, J., Mitchell, D., Smiciklas-Wright, H., & Birch, L. (2002). Parental influences on young girls' fruit and vegetable, micronutrient, and fat intakes. *Journal of the American Dietetic Association*, 102(1), 58-64.

Gantz, W., Schwartz, N., Angelini, J., & Rideout, V. Henry Kaiser Family Foundation, (2007). *Food for thought: Television food advertising to children in the United States*. Retrieved from website: http://www.kff.org/entmedia/upload/7618.pdf

Gustafson-Larson, A., & Terry, R. (1992). Weight-related behaviors and concerns of fourth-grade children. *Journal of the American Dietetic Association*, 92(7), 818-822.

International Food Information Council Foundation, (2008). *IFIC Review: Breakfast and Health*. Retrieved from website: http://bit.ly/y9VUrg

McCabe, M., & Ricciardelli, L. (2001). Parent, peer, and media influences on body image and strategies to both increase and decrease body size among adolescent boys and girls. *Adolescence*, 36(142), 225-240.

McGinnis, J. M., Gootman, J., & A., Kraak, V. I., eds. (2006). *Food marketing to children and youth, threat or opportunity?* Natl Academy Pr. Retrieved from http://www.iom.edu/Reports/2005/Food-Marketing-to-Children-and-Youth-Threat-or-Opportunity.aspx

McLellan, F. (2002). Marketing and advertising: harmful to children's health. *Lancet*, 360(9338), 1001.

Mellin, L., Irwin, C., & Scully, S. (1992). Prevalence of disordered eating in girls: a survey of middle-class children. *Journal of the American Dietetic Association*, 92(7), 851-853.

Neumark-Sztainer, D., Sherwood, N., Coller, T., & Hannan, P. (2000). Primary prevention of disordered eating among preadolescent girls: feasibility and short-term effect of a community-based intervention. *Journal of the American Dietetic Association*, 100(12), 1466-1473.

Pierce, J., & Wardle, J. (1993). Self-esteem, parental appraisal and body size in children. *Journal of Child Psychology and Psychiatry, and Allied Disciplines*, 34(7), 1125-1136.

Rampersaud, G., Pereira, M., Girard, B., Adams, J., & Metzl, J. (2005). Breakfast habits, nutritional status, body weight, and academic performance in children and adolescents. *Journal of the American Dietetic Association*, 105(5), 743-760.

Rideout, V., Foehr, U., & Roberts, D. The Kaiser Family Foundation, (2010). *Generation M2: Media in the Lives of 8- to 18-Year-Olds*. Retrieved from website: http://www.kff.org/entmedia/upload/8010.pdf

Robinson, T. (1999). Reducing children's television viewing to prevent obesity: a randomized controlled trial. JAMA: *The Journal of The American Medical Association*, 282(16), 1561-1567.

U.S. Department of Agriculture and U.S. Department of Health and Human Services, (2011). *Dietary Guidelines for Americans, 2010. 7th edition*. Retrieved from website: http://www.cnpp.usda.gov/DietaryGuidelines.htm

U.S. Department of Agriculture. (2012). *ChooseMyPlate.gov Website*. Washington, DC.

U.S. Department of Health and Human Services Office on Women's health (2009). *Body image and your kids*. Retrieved from website: http://www.womenshealth.gov/body-image/kids/

van den Berg, P., Neumark-Sztainer, D., Hannan, P., & Haines, J. (2007). Is dieting advice from magazines helpful or harmful? Five-year associations with weight-control behaviors and psychological outcomes in adolescents. *Pediatrics*, 119(1), e30-e37.

CHAPTER 3

Brener, N., Chriqui, J., O'Toole, T., Schwartz, M., & McManus, T. (2011). Establishing a baseline measure of school wellness-related policies implemented in a nationally representative sample of school districts. *Journal of the American Dietetic Association*, 111(6), 894-901.

Briggs, M., Mueller, C., & Fleischhacker, S. (2010). Position of the American Dietetic Association, School Nutrition Association, and Society for Nutrition Education: comprehensive school nutrition services. *Journal of the American Dietetic Association*, 110(11), 1738-1749.

Contento, I. (2008). Nutrition education: linking research, theory, and practice. *Asia Pacific Journal of Clinical Nutrition*, 17 Suppl 1176-179.

Fleischhacker, S., Schure, J., Contento, I., Freier, L., Fox, T., Mosack, J., & Soltanmora, K. Society for Nutrition Education, (2009). *State of nutrition education & promotion for children & adolescents*. Retrieved from website: http://bit.ly/zVfEN5

Florence, M., Asbridge, M., & Veugelers, P. (2008). Diet quality and academic performance. The *Journal of School Health*, 78(4), 209-215.

Foster, G., Sherman, S., Borradaile, K., Grundy, K., Vander Veur, S., Nachmani, J., & ... Shults, J. (2008). A policy-based school intervention to prevent overweight and obesity. *Pediatrics*, 121(4), e794-e802. Retrieved from http://pediatrics.aappublications.org/content/121/4/e794.full

Hammerschmidt, P., Tackett, W., Golzynski, M., & Golzynski, D. (2011). Barriers to and facilitators of healthful eating and physical activity in low-income schools. *Journal of Nutrition Education and Behavior*, 43(1), 63-68.

Hearn, M., Baranowski, T., Baranowski, J., Doyle, C., Smith, M., Lin, L., & Resnicow, K. (1998). Environmental influences on dietary behavior among children: availability and accessibility of fruits and vegetables enable consumption. *Journal of Health Education*, 29, 26-32.

Kelder, S.H., Perry, C.L., Klepp, K., & Lytle, L.L. (1994). Longitudinal tracking of adolescent smoking, physical activity, and food choice behaviors. *American Journal of Public Health*, 84, 1121-1126.

Kristjansdottir, A., Johannsson, E., & Thorsdottir, I. (2010). Effects of a school-based intervention on adherence of 7-9-year-olds to food-based dietary guidelines and intake of nutrients. *Public Health Nutrition*, 13(8), 1151-1161.

Liquori, T., Koch, P. D., Contento, I. R., & Castle, J. (1998). The cookshop program: Outcome evaluation of a nutrition education program linking lunchroom food experiences with classroom cooking components. *Journal of Nutrition Education*, 30, 302-313

Lytle, L. (1995). Nutrition education for school-aged children. *Journal of Nutrition Education*, 27(6), 298-311.

Murphy, A., Youatt, J., Hoerr, S., Sawyer, C., & Andrews, S. (1994). Nutrition education needs and learning preferences of Michigan students in grades 5, 8, and 11. *The Journal of School Health*, 64(7), 273-278.

Nader, P., Stone, E., Lytle, L., Perry, C., Osganian, S., Kelder, S., & ... Luepker, R. (1999). Three-year maintenance of improved diet and physical activity: the CATCH cohort. Child and Adolescent Trial for Cardiovascular Health. *Archives of Pediatrics & Adolescent Medicine*, 153(7), 695-704.

Pérez-Escamilla, R., Haldeman, L., & Gray, S. (2002). Assessment of nutrition education needs in an urban school district in Connecticut: establishing priorities through research. *Journal of the American Dietetic Association*, 102(4), 559-562.

Perry, C. L., Bishop, D. B., Taylor, G., Murray, D. M., Mays, R. W., Dudovitz, B. S., et al. (1998). Changing fruit and vegetable consumption among children: The 5-a-Day power plus program in St. Paul, Minnesota. *American Journal of Public Health*, 88, 603-609.

Rideout, V., Foehr, U., & Roberts, D. The Kaiser Family Foundation, (2010). *Generation M2: Media in the Lives of 8- to 18-Year-Olds*. Retrieved from website: http://www.kff.org/entmedia/upload/8010.pdf

Roseman, M., Riddell, M., & Haynes, J. (2011). A content analysis of kindergarten-12th grade school-based nutrition interventions: taking advantage of past learning. *Journal of Nutrition Education and Behavior*, 43(1), 2-18.

Thomas, L., Long, E., & Zaske, J. (1994). Nutrition education sources and priorities of elementary school teachers. Journal of the American Dietetic Association, 94(3), 318-320.

U.S. Department of Agriculture. *Healthy hunger-free kids act of 2010*. Retrieved from http://www.fns.usda.gov/cnd/governance/legislation/CNR_2010.htm

U.S. Department of Education, National Center for Education Statistics, (2000). *Nutrition education in public elementary school classrooms*. NCES 2000-040. Retrieved from website: http://nces.ed.gov/pubs2000/2000040.pdf

CHAPTER 4

Carlson, A., Mancino, L., & Lino, M. United States Department of Agriculture , Center for Nutrition Policy and Promotion. (2005). *Grain consumption by Americans*. Retrieved from website: http://1.usa.gov/ydikA8

Hasler, C., & Brown, A. (2009). Position of the American Dietetic Association: functional foods. *Journal of the American Dietetic Association*, 109(4), 735-746.

International Food Information Council Foundation, (2011). *Functional foods*. Retrieved from website: http://bit.ly/wApyim

O'Neil, C., Nicklas, T., Zanovec, M., Cho, S., & Kleinman, R. (2011). Consumption of whole grains is associated with improved diet quality and nutrient intake in children and adolescents: the National Health and Nutrition Examination Survey 1999-2004. *Public Health Nutrition*, 14(2), 347-355.

U.S. Department of Agriculture and U.S. Department of Health and Human Services, (2011). *Dietary Guidelines for Americans, 2010. 7th edition*. Retrieved from website: http://www.cnpp.usda.gov/DietaryGuidelines.htm

U.S. Department of Agriculture. (2012). *ChooseMyPlate.gov Website*. Washington, DC.

Children's books:

Conford, E. (2006). *What's Cooking, Jenny Archer?* Little, Brown Young Readers.

Herman, D. & Bailey, S. (2004). *Carla's Sandwich*. Flashlight Press.

CHAPTER 5

U.S. Department of Agriculture. (2012). *ChooseMyPlate.gov Website*. Washington, DC.

Corporation for Public Broadcasting. (2004). *Don't buy it: Get media smart*. Retrieved from website: http://pbskids.org/dontbuyit

Children's books:

Berenstain, S. & Berenstain, J. (1985). *The Berenstain Bears and Too Much Junk Food*. New York: Random House.

Brown, M. (1986). *Stone Soup*. New York: Aladdin Books.

Browne, E. (1999). *Handa's surprise*. Cambridge, Mass: Candlewick Press.

Butterworth, C. & Gaggiotti, L. (2011). *How Did That Get in My Lunchbox? The Story of Food*. Somerville, Mass: Candlewick Press.

Charney, S., Goldbeck, D. & Larson, M. (2007). *The ABCs of Fruits and Vegetables and beyond*. Woodstock: Ceres Press.

Child, L. (2003). I *will never not ever eat a tomato*. Cambridge, Mass: Candlewick Press.

Conford, E. (2006). *What's Cooking, Jenny Archer*? Little, Brown Young Readers.

Coy, J. & Fisher, C. (2009). *Two Old Potatoes and Me*. New York: Dragonfly Books.

DeClements, B. (2009). *Nothing's fair in fifth grade*. New York, N.Y: Puffin Books.

Diakite, B. (1999). *The Hatseller and the Monkeys*. New York: Scholastic Press.

Evers, C. & Disney Artists (2006). *Good for You! Nutrition Book and Games*. New York: Disney Press.

Ehlert, L. (1993). *Eating the Alphabet*. San Diego: Voyager Books.

French, V. (1998). *Oliver's fruit salad*. London: Hodder Children's.

French, V. & Bartlett, A. (2000). *Oliver's Milkshake*. London: Hodder Children's Books.

French, V. (1996). *Oliver's vegetables*. S. l: Orchard.

Gibbons, G. (2008). *The Vegetables We Eat*. New York: Holiday House.

Grigsby, S. (2010). *In the garden with Doctor Carver*. Chicago, Ill: Albert Whitman.

Hoban, R. & Hoban, L. (2008). *Bread and Jam for Frances*. London: HarperCollins. (reissued edition)

Mccloskey, R. (2010). *Blueberries for Sal*. London: Puffin. (reissued edition)

Miller, E. (2006). *The Monster Health Book*. New York: Holiday House.

Ottolenghi, C. (2002). *The little red hen*. Columbus, Ohio: McGraw-Hill Children's Pub.

Park, B. (2003). *Junie B., first grader: boss of lunch*. New York: Scholastic.

Pollan, M. (2009). *The omnivore's dilemma for kids: the secrets behind what you eat*. New York: Dial Books.

Sayre, A. (2011). *Rah, rah, radishes! : a vegetable chant*. New York: Beach Lane Books.

Shanley, E. & Thompson, C. (2011). *Fueling the teen machine : what it takes to make good choices for yourself every day*. Boulder, Colo: Bull Pub. Co.

Seuss, D. (1960). *Green eggs and ham*. New York: Random House, Inc.

Storper, B. (2011). *Janey Junkfood's fresh adventure! Making Good Eating Great Fun!* Hatfield, MA: FoodPlay Productions.

Sturges, P. (2002). *The little red hen (makes a pizza)*. New York: Puffin Books.

CHAPTER 6

Johnson, R., Appel, L., Brands, M., Howard, B., Lefevre, M., Lustig, R., & ... Wylie-Rosett, J. (2009). Dietary sugars intake and cardiovascular health: a scientific statement from the American Heart Association. *Circulation*, 120(11), 1011-1020.

U.S. Department of Agriculture and U.S. Department of Health and Human Services, (2011). *Dietary Guidelines for Americans, 2010. 7th edition.* Retrieved from website: http://www.cnpp.usda.gov/DietaryGuidelines.htm

U.S. Department of Agriculture. (2012).*ChooseMyPlate.gov Website.* Washington, DC.

U.S. Food and Drug Administration. (2011). *Nutrition facts label programs and materials.* Retrieved from http://www.fda.gov/Food/ResourcesForYou/Consumers/NFLPM.

CHAPTER 7

Davis, J., Ventura, E., Cook, L., Gyllenhammer, L., & Gatto, N. (2011). LA Sprouts: a gardening, nutrition, and cooking intervention for Latino youth improves diet and reduces obesity. *Journal of the American Dietetic Association,* 111(8), 1224-1230.

Getlinger, M., Laughlin, V., Bell, E., Akre, C., & Arjmandi, B. (1996). Food waste is reduced when elementary-school children have recess before lunch. *Journal of the American Dietetic Association,* 96(9), 906-908.

International Food Information Council Foundation, (2008). *IFIC Review: Breakfast and Health.* Retrieved from website: http://bit.ly/y9VUrg

Lu, C., Toepel, K., Irish, R., Fenske, R., Barr, D., & Bravo, R. (2006). Organic diets significantly lower children's dietary exposure to organophosphorus pesticides. *Environmental Health Perspectives* 114(2): 260-3.

Morris, J., Koumjian, K., Briggs, M., & Zidenberg-Cherr, S. (2002). Nutrition to grow on: a garden-enhanced nutrition education curriculum for upper-elementary schoolchildren. *Journal of Nutrition Education and Behavior,* 34(3), 175-176.

Patten, E. (2003). *Healthy foods from healthy soils: a hands-on resource for educato*rs. Gardner, Me: Tilbury House Publishers.

Rampersaud, G., Pereira, M., Girard, B., Adams, J., & Metzl, J. (2005). Breakfast habits, nutritional status, body weight, and academic performance in children and adolescents. *Journal of the American Dietetic Association*, 105(5), 743-760.

Robinson-O'Brien, R., Story, M., & Heim, S. (2009). Impact of garden-based youth nutrition intervention programs: A review. *Journal of the American Dietetic Association*, 109, 273-280.

Sizer, F. & Whitney, E. (2012). *Nutrition Concepts and Controversies, MyPlate Update*. Brooks/Cole Pub Co.

Smith, D. & Margolskee, R. (2001). Making sense of taste. *Scientific American*, 284 (3): 32–9.

U.S. Department of Agriculture and U.S. Department of Health and Human Services, (2011). *Dietary Guidelines for Americans, 2010. 7th edition*. Retrieved from website: http://www.cnpp.usda.gov/DietaryGuidelines.htm

U.S. Department of Agriculture, Agricultural Research Service. (2012). *USDA National Nutrient Database for Standard Reference, Release 24*. Retrieved from website: http://www.ars.usda.gov/Services/docs.htm?docid=8964

U.S. Department of Health & Human Services, (n.d.). Sprouts: What you should know. Retrieved from website: http://www.foodsafety.gov/keep/types/fruits/sprouts.html

Children's Books:

Cherry, L. (2003). *How Groundhog's Garden Grew*. New York: Blue Sky Press.

Coy, J. & Fisher, C. (2009). *Two Old Potatoes and Me*. New York: Dragonfly Books.

Epstein, S. (1978). *Dr. Beaumont and the man with the hole in his stomach*. New York: Coward, McCann & Geoghegan.

Gibbons, G. (2008). *The Vegetables We Eat.* New York: Holiday House.

Grigsby, S. (2010). *In the garden with Doctor Carver.* Chicago, Ill: Albert Whitman.

Grigsby, S. (2012). *First peas to the table: how Thomas Jefferson inspired a school garden.* Chicago, Ill: Albert Whitman.

Milway, K. & Daigneault, S. (2010). *Good Garden, The: How One Family Went from Hunger to Having Enough.* Toronto: Kids Can Press.

Nagro, A. (2011). *Our super garden: learning the power of healthy eating, by eating what we grow.* United States: Dancing Rhinoceros Press.

Showers, P. (2001). *What happens to a hamburger.* New York: HarperCollins.

Swanson, D. (2001). *Burp!: the most interesting book you'll ever read about eating.* Toronto: Kids Can Press.

CHAPTER 8

Albala, K. (2007). *Beans: a history.* Oxford New York: Berg.

Coleman-Jenson, A., Nord, M., Andrews, G., & Carlson, S. (2011). *Household food security in the united states in 2010.* Retrieved from website: http://www.ers.usda.gov/Publications/err125/

D'Aluisio, F. & Menzel, P. (2008). *What the world eats.* Berkeley, Calif: Tricycle Press.

Frank, L. (2002). *Foods of the Southwest Indian nations : traditional & contemporary Native American recipes.* Berkeley, Calif: Ten Speed Press.

Fussell, B. (2004). *The story of corn.* Albuquerque: University of New Mexico Press.

Hartline-Grafton, H. (2011). *Food insecurity and obesity: Understanding the connections.* Food Research and Action Center. Retrieved from http://frac.org/pdf/frac_brief_understanding_the_connections.pdf

Mintz, S. (1993). *Feeding, eating, and grazing: some speculations on modern food habits.* Journal of Gastronomy. 7:46-57.

Project EAT. (n.d.). *Project results.* University of Minnesota School of Public Health. Retrieved from http://www.sph.umn.edu/epi/research/eat/results.asp

U.S. Department of Agriculture, National Agricultural Library. (n.d.). *Ethnic and Cultural Resources: Dietary Guidelines from Around the World.* Retrieved from website: http://www.nal.usda.gov/

U.S. Department of Agriculture. (2012). *ChooseMyPlate.gov Website.* Washington, DC.

Children's Books:

Aliki. (1986). Corn *is maize, the gift of the Indians.* HarperCollins.

Amico, J. & Drummond, K. (2005). *The coming to America cookbook : Delicious recipes and fascinating stories from America's many cultures.* Hoboken, N.J: Wiley.

Browne, E. (1999). *Handa's surprise.* Cambridge, Mass: Candlewick Press.

Cook, D. (2008). *The kids' multicultural cookbook : food & fun from around the world.* Nashville, Tenn: Williamson Books.

Cutler, J. (2011). *Family dinner.* Bloomington, IN: iUniverse, Inc.

Diakite, B. (1999). *The Hatseller and the Monkeys.* New York: Scholastic Press.

Dodge, A. (2008). *Around the world cookbook.* New York: DK Publishing.

Dooley, N. (1996). *Everybody bakes bread.* Minneapolis: Carolrhoda Books.

Dooley, N. (1996). *Everybody cooks rice.* Boston: Houghton Mifflin.

Dooley, N. (2004). *Everybody serves soup.* Minneapolis: First Avenue Editions.

Friedman, I. & Say, A. (1987). *How My Parents Learned to Eat*. Boston: Houghton Mifflin.

Gershator, D. (1998). *Bread is for eating*. New York: H. Holt.

Gibbons, G. (2008). *Corn*. New York: Holiday House.

Grigsby, S. (2010). In *the garden with Doctor Carver*. Chicago, Ill: Albert Whitman.

Hester, D. (2007). *Grandma Lena's big ol' turnip*. Morton Grove, Ill: Albert Whitman & Co.

Lauber, P., & Manders, J. (2009). *What You Never Knew About Fingers, Forks and Chopsticks*. New York: Simon & Schuster Books for Young Readers.

Lin, G. (1999). *The ugly vegetables*. Watertown, MA: Charlesbridge.

Milway, K. & Daigneault, S. (2010). *Good Garden, The: How One Family Went from Hunger to Having Enough*. Toronto: Kids Can Press.

Mora, P. (2007). *Yum! mmmm! qué rico! : Americas' sproutings*. New York: Lee & Low Books Inc.

Webb, L. (2009). *The multicultural cookbook for students*. Santa Barbara, CA: Greenwood Press.

Weiss, E. (2008). *From kernel to corncob*. Danbury, Conn: Children's Press.

CHAPTER 9

Burstein, J. (2008). *Big fat lies: advertising tricks*. New York: Crabtree Publishing Co.

Gantz, W., Schwartz, N., Angelini, J., & Rideout, V. Henry Kaiser Family Foundation, (2007). *Food for thought: Television food advertising to children in the United States*. Retrieved from website: http://www.kff.org/entmedia/upload/7618.pdf

McGinnis, J. M., Gootman, J., & A., Kraak, V. I., eds. (2006). *Food marketing to children and youth, threat or opportunity?* Natl Academy Pr. Retrieved from http://bit.ly/wvPkWC

Neumark-Sztainer, D., Haines, J., Robinson-O'Brien, R., Hannan, P., Robins, M., Morris, B., & Petrich, C. (2009). *'Ready. Set. ACTION!' A theater-based obesity prevention program for children: a feasibility study.* Health Education Research, 24(3), 407-420.

Nicklas, T., Goh, E., Goodell, L., Acuff, D., Reiher, R., Buday, R., & Ottenbacher, A. (2011). *Impact of commercials on food preferences of low-income, minority preschoolers.* Journal of Nutrition Education and Behavior, 43(1), 35-41.

Perry, C., Zauner, M., Oakes, J., Taylor, G., & Bishop, D. (2002). *Evaluation of a theater production about eating behavior of children.* The Journal Of School Health, 72(6), 256-261.

Rideout, V., Foehr, U., & Roberts, D. The Kaiser Family Foundation, (2010). *Generation M2: Media in the Lives of 8- to 18-Year-Olds.* Retrieved from website: http://www.kff.org/entmedia/upload/8010.pdf

CHAPTER 10

Chefs move to schools. (n.d.). Retrieved from http://www.chefsmovetoschools.org/

Elffers, J. & Freymann, S. (2006). *Fast food.* New York: Arthur A. Levine Books.

U.S. Department of Health & Human Services, (n.d.). *Sprouts: What you should know.* Retrieved from website: http://www.foodsafety.gov/keep/types/fruits/sprouts.html

CHAPTER 11

Blom, L., Alvarez, J., Zhang, L., & Kolbo, J. (2011). Associations between health-related physical fitness, academic achievement and selected academic behaviors of elementary and middle school students in the state of Mississippi. *ICHPER-SD Journal of Research*, 6(1), 13-19. Retrieved from http://20.132.48.254/PDFS/EJ936015.pdf

Centers for Disease Control and Prevention, U.S. Department of Health and Human Services. (2010). *The association between school based physical activity, including physical education, and academic performance.* Retrieved from website: http://1.usa.gov/A2gD19

Crespo, C., Smit, E., Troiano, R., Bartlett, S., Macera, C., & Andersen, R. (2001). Television watching, energy intake, and obesity in US children: results from the third National Health and Nutrition Examination Survey, 1988-1994. *Archives of Pediatrics & Adolescent Medicine*, 155(3), 360-365.

Fox, C., Barr-Anderson, D., Neumark-Sztainer, D., & Wall, M. (2010). Physical activity and sports team participation: associations with academic outcomes in middle school and high school students. The *Journal of School Health*, 80(1), 31-37.

Hopper, C., Fisher, B., & Munoz, K. (2008). *Physical activity and nutrition for health.* Champaign, IL: Human Kinetics.

Johnson C. (1989). *Taking the classroom beyond four walls.* Newsletter of Oregon Association of the Advancement of Health Education (OAAHE).

Knoflach, M., Kiechl, S., Kind, M., Said, M., Sief, R., Gisinger, M., & ... Wick, G. (2003). Cardiovascular risk factors and atherosclerosis in young males: ARMY study (Atherosclerosis Risk-Factors in Male Youngsters). *Circulation*, 108(9), 1064-1069.

Lets move! America's Move to Raise a Healthier Generation of Kids. (2010). Retrieved from http://www.letsmove.gov/

McGill, H., McMahan, C., Zieske, A., Sloop, G., Walcott, J., Troxclair, D., & ... Strong, J. (2000). Associations of coronary heart disease risk factors with the intermediate lesion of atherosclerosis in youth. The Pathobiological Determinants of Atherosclerosis in Youth (PDAY) Research Group. *Arteriosclerosis, Thrombosis, and Vascular Biology*, 20(8), 1998-2004.

Nader, P., Bradley, R., Houts, R., McRitchie, M., & O'Brien, M. (2008). Moderate-to-vigorous physical activity from ages 9 to 15 years. *Journal of the American Medical Association*, 300(3), 295-305. Retrieved from http://jama.ama-assn.org/content/300/3/295.full.pdf

U.S. Department of Agriculture and U.S. Department of Health and Human Services. (2011). *Dietary Guidelines for Americans, 2010. 7th edition*. Retrieved from website: http://www.cnpp.usda.gov/DietaryGuidelines.htm

U.S. Department of Agriculture. (2012). *ChooseMyPlate.gov Website*. Washington, DC.

U.S. Department of Health and Human Services, Office of Disease Prevention and Health Promotion. (2008). *2008 Physical Activity Guidelines for Americans*. Publication No. U0036. Retrieved from website: http://www.health.gov/paguidelines

CHAPTER 12

Briggs, M., Mueller, C., & Fleischhacker, S. (2010). Position of the American Dietetic Association, School Nutrition Association, and Society for Nutrition Education: comprehensive school nutrition services. *Journal of the American Dietetic Association*, 110(11), 1738-1749.

Cornell Food & Brand Lab. (2011) Eat Your Vegetables: Preschoolers Love Vegetables With Catchy Names Like 'X-Ray Vision Carrots' And 'Tomato Bursts'. *ScienceDaily*, 4 Mar. 2009. Retrieved from website: http://www.sciencedaily.com/releases/2009/03/090302120019.htm

Cornell University Food and Brand Lab. (n.d.). *Smarter lunchrooms movement: Food's not nutrition until it's eaten*. Retrieved from http://smarterlunchrooms.org

Evers C. (1995). More nutrition, less waste. *School Foodservice & Nutrition*, November:76.

Evers C. (2000). A nutrition education report card. *School Foodservice & Nutrition*, June/July:22-30.

Foster, G., Sherman, S., Borradaile, K., Grundy, K., Vander Veur, S., Nachmani, J., & ... Shults, J. (2008). A policy-based school intervention to prevent overweight and obesity. *Pediatrics*, 121(4), e794-e802. Retrieved from http://pediatrics.aappublications.org/content/121/4/e794.full

Harding Lawson Associates. (1994). *Offer Versus Serve and Food Choices in Elementary School Cafeterias: Waste Prevention Pilot Projects at North Plains Elementary School, Charles F. Tigard Elementary School, and Metzger Elementary School*, Unpublished report.

Healthy hunger-free kids act of 2010. Retrieved from http://www.fns.usda.gov/cnd/governance/legislation/CNR_2010.htm

Kubik, M., Lytle, L., & Story, M. (2001). A practical, theory-based approach to establishing school nutrition advisory councils. *Journal of the American Dietetic Association*, 101(2), 223-228.

Lets move! America's Move to Raise a Healthier Generation of Kids. (2010). Retrieved from http://www.letsmove.gov/

Schwartz, M. (2007). The influence of a verbal prompt on school lunch fruit consumption: a pilot study. *International Journal of Behavioral Nutrition and Physical Activity*, 4:6.

Story, M. (2009). The third School Nutrition Dietary Assessment Study: findings and policy implications for improving the health of US children. *Journal of the American Dietetic Association*, 109(2 Suppl), S7-S13.

Turner, L., & Chaloupka, F. (2012). Student access to competitive foods in elementary schools: trends over time and regional differences. *Archives of Pediatrics & Adolescent Medicine*, 166(2), 164-169.

Turner, L., Chaloupka, F. & Sandoval, A. (2012). *School Policies and Practices for Improving Children's Health: National Elementary School Survey Results: School Years 2006–07 through 2009–10. Vol. 2.* Robert Wood Johnson Foundation, Bridging the Gap. Retrieved from website: http://www.bridgingthegapresearch.org

U.S. Department of Agriculture and U.S. Department of Health and Human Services, (2011). *Dietary Guidelines for Americans, 2010. 7th edition.* Retrieved from website: http://www.cnpp.usda.gov/DietaryGuidelines.htm

U.S. Department of Agriculture. (2012). *ChooseMyPlate.gov Website.* Washington, DC.

Index

Made in the USA
Lexington, KY
15 March 2016